ABC OF ASTHMA

ABC OF ASTHMA

THIRD EDITION

JOHN REES MD FRCP
Senior lecturer and consultant physician,
Guy's Hospital

and

JOHN PRICE MD FRCP DCH
Professor and consultant paediatrician,
King's College Hospital

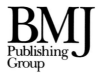

© BMJ Publishing Group 1984, 1989, 1995

First edition 1984
Second edition 1984
Second impression 1991
Third impression 1992
Third edition 1995
Second impression 1996

British Library Cataloguing in Publication Data

A catalogue record for this book is available from the British Library

ISBN 0-7279-0882-0

Typeset by Apek Typesetters Limited, Nailsea, Bristol
Printed in Great Britain by Thanet Press Limited, Margate

Contents

ACKNOWLEDGEMENTS

The graphs on pages 2, 4, 10, 11, 20, 27, 34, 35, 36, and 38 were based on data from the following papers; Peak JK, *et al*, *BMJ* 1994;**308**:1591–6; Miller RD, *et al*, *Thorax* 1992;**47**:904–9; Waite DA, *et al*, *Clinical Allergy* 1980;**10**:71–5; Shapiro C, ed. *ABC of Sleep Disorders*, London: BMJ, 1993:52; Gregg I, *et al*, *BMJ* 1989;**298**:1068–70; Ullman *et al*, *Thorax* 1988;**43**:674–8; D'Alonzo D, *et al*, *Am Rev Respir Dis* 1990;**142**:84–90; Anderson HR, *Pediatric Respiratory Medicine* 1993;**1**:6–10; Weitzman M, *et al*, *Pediatrics* 1990;**85**:505–11; Dold *et al*, *Arch Dis Child* 1992;**67**:1018–22; Crane *et al*, *J All Clin Immunol* 1989;**84**:768.

The pictures of the boy with the snowman by Keith Barnard (p 1), the girl practising yoga (p 15), the girl smoking by Richard Gardner (p 25), apple blossom by TH Williams (p 30), and the woman using a vacuum cleaner by Day Williams (p 42) are copyright Barnaby's Picture Library; the woman with a buggy crossing the street (p 16), the girls running (p 41), and the children running (p 42) are copyright Ulrike Preuss; the house dust mite (p 13) is copyright David Scharf/Science Photo Library; the pregnant woman (p 16) is copyright John Rae; *Atropa belladonna* (p 22) is copyright Heather Angel; and the nurse with the baby (p 41) is copyright Hank Morgan/Science Picture Library. The pictures of food allergens (p 14), "Snoopy" (p 30), and "Ben" (p 41), were taken by Mary Evans. The electron microscope picture of pollen grains reproduced on the cover and p 36 was taken by R Whitenstall, Department of Materials, Queen Mary and Westfield College.

DEFINITION AND DIAGNOSIS

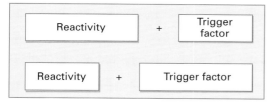

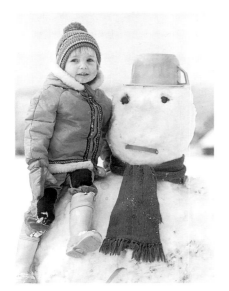

Cold air is a stimulus for asthma.

Asthma is a common condition which, despite the attention it has received during the last few years, is still underdiagnosed and undertreated. Moderately severe asthma with attacks of wheezing that are precipitated by specific stimuli is relatively easy to recognise, but there may be difficulties with more severe disease when lung function never returns completely to normal between attacks. In mild cases obstruction of airflow may be intermittent with no symptoms of asthma between events.

The clinical characteristic of asthma is airflow obstruction, which can be reversed over short periods of time or with treatment. This may be evident from provocation by specific stimuli or from the response to bronchodilator drugs.

A commonly used definition of asthma is: a disease characterised by wide variations over short periods of time in resistance to airflow in intrapulmonary airways. Other definitions have been used, some of which include the necessity to show airway hyper-responsiveness to stimuli such as methacholine or histamine. For example, the International Consensus Report on the Diagnosis and Management of Asthma (*Clin Exper Allergy* 1992; **22** suppl 1) reads:

> Asthma is a chronic inflammatory disorder of the airways in which many cells play a role, including mast cells and eosinophils. In susceptible individuals this inflammation causes symptoms which are usually associated with widespread but variable airflow obstruction that is often reversible either spontaneously or with treatment, and causes an associated increase in airway responsiveness to a variety of stimuli.

Most asthmatics develop narrowing of the airways in response to small amounts of these agents and, in general, the more severe the asthma the more the airways react on challenge. Other stimuli such as cold air, exercise, and hypotonic solutions can also provoke this increased reactivity. In contrast, it is difficult to induce significant narrowing of the airways with many of these stimuli in healthy people. In some epidemiological studies increased airway responsiveness is used as part of the definition of asthma. Wheezing during the past 12 months is added to exclude those who have increased responsiveness but no symptoms.

In clinical practice in the United Kingdom airway responsiveness demonstrated in the laboratory is rarely used in the diagnosis of asthma. The clinical equivalent of symptoms in response to dust, smoke, cold air, and exercise should be sought in the history.

In the past there was a tendency to use the term "wheezy bronchitis" in children rather than asthma in the belief that this would protect the parents from the label of asthma. In adults who smoke it may be difficult to differentiate from the airway narrowing that is part of chronic bronchitis and emphysema that have been caused by previous cigarette smoking.

The actual diagnostic label would not matter if the appropriate treatment was used. Unfortunately the evidence shows that children who are diagnosed as having asthma are more likely to get appropriate prophylaxis than children with the same symptoms who are given an

Definition and diagnosis

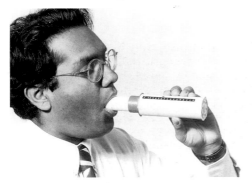

Portable peak flow meters are useful in the diagnosis and monitoring of asthma.

alternative "label". In adults attempts at bronchodilatation and prophylaxis are more extensive in those who are labelled as asthmatic. Asthma is such a common and well publicised condition now that it is best to accept the diagnosis when it is appropriate, to explain the implications to patients and parents, and to begin the correct treatment. Persistent problems of cough and wheeze are likely to be much more worrying than the correct diagnosis and improvement in symptoms on treatment. The particular problems of the diagnosis of asthma in very young children will be dealt with in chapter 10.

In older patients with any form of widespread airflow obstruction it is appropriate to try to achieve adequate bronchodilatation which should be confirmed by objective testing. Prophylaxis with inhaled corticosteroids is well established as an important part of the treatment of asthma. There are some indications that the same treatment could slow the rate of decline of lung function in patients with chronic bronchitis and emphysema. If this is true then the approach to treatment of the two conditions will be similar and the drug bill for inhaled corticosteroids will increase greatly.

Prevalence

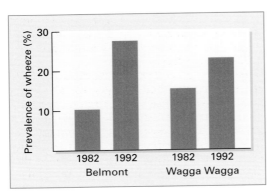

Increase in prevalence of wheeze in 8–10 year old children in two towns in New South Wales between 1982 and 1992. There was a pronounced increase in counts of house dust mite in domestic dust over the same period.

The reported prevalence depends on the definition of asthma being used, and the age and type of the population being studied. Although changes in criteria and fashions make interpretation difficult a number of studies have suggested that there is a slow increase in the prevalence of asthma in most countries. There are regional variations, particularly among developing countries in which the rates in urban areas are higher than in the poor rural districts. In developed countries there is no association with social class except a tendency to give the label of asthma more readily to those in social classes I and II.

In the United States asthma is more prevalent among blacks than whites but in the UK the association is less pronounced. Asians have a lower prevalence than whites in the UK.

In children the prevalence of asthma in the 5–12 year age group is over 10%. Australian studies give a prevalence nearer 20%. The sex ratio in children around 7 years shows that one and a half to twice as many boys are affected as girls, but during their teenage years boys do better than girls and by the time they reach adulthood the sex incidence has become about equal.

Wheezing is a common symptom, and questionnaires have shown that about 30% of the population wheezes at some time. In many cases the wheezing is temporary and develops after a viral infection in otherwise normal subjects. The inflammation of the airway leaves nerve endings exposed and vulnerable to the effects of potentially harmful stimuli such as smoke and dust particles.

Most studies that have used equivalent diagnostic criteria in a stable group have suggested that the prevalence is increasing. This is more difficult to judge in young children and in subjects over 50 years old when differential diagnoses produce uncertainty. The results fit in with other information such as the data on general practitioners' workload with asthmatic patients.

Genetics

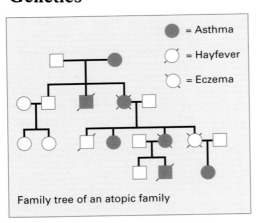

Family tree of an atopic family

There is a familial link in asthma; in the island of Tristan da Cunha, for example, a high prevalence of asthma can be traced back to three asthmatic women among the original settlers. There are also associations with other atopic disorders such as rhinitis and eczema. More recently atopy has been linked to the maternal 11q13 allele, suggesting inheritance of atopy through the chromosome 11q locus from the mother. This has not been confirmed by all workers, but may be the genetic explanation in some groups of patients. The results are likely to depend on the selection of the group to be tested. Although these results are debatable they are the first inkling of a chromosomal site for an atopic gene. This raises the possibility of useful treatment in the future based around the genetic abnormality, but such speculation takes us a long time into the future.

Pathology

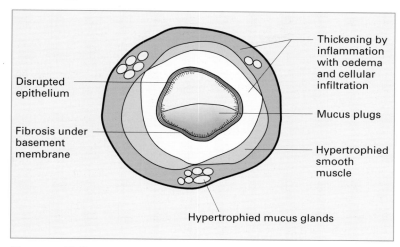

Thickening by inflammation with oedema and cellular infiltration

Disrupted epithelium

Fibrosis under basement membrane

Mucus plugs

Hypertrophied smooth muscle

Hypertrophied mucus glands

Diagram of inflammatory changes in the airway.

The wall of the airway in asthma is thickened by oedema, cellular infiltration, increased smooth muscle and glands. There is an infiltration by numerous cells, particularly neutrophils and eosinophils, but also lymphocytes and a few mast cells. Lymphocytes may be the source of the messengers, interleukins which attract polymorphonuclear cells which then release compounds which cause further local inflammation and damage. The basement membrane or the tissue just beneath it becomes thickened. The damage to the wall may lead to scarring and persistent narrowing of the airway, which loses its ability to respond completely to bronchodilators.

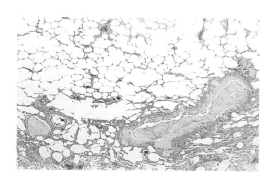

Plugged airways in asthma.

In severe asthma there is mucus plugging within the lumen and loss of parts of the surface epithelium. Extensive mucus plugging is the striking finding in the lungs of patients who die of an acute exacerbation of asthma.

In patients with mild asthma who have largely been free of symptoms for months there is still evidence of inflammation in the wall of the airway. This suggests that the underlying susceptibility is still present and will reappear given the suitable stimulus.

It has been suggested that asthma is a generalised abnormality of the inflammatory or immune cells and that the lungs are just the site where the symptoms show. This does not explain the recent finding that lungs from a patient with mild asthma transplanted into a normal donor produced problems with obstruction of airflow while normal lungs transplanted in to an asthmatic patient were free of problems. It seems that the immunological abnormality that provokes inflammation of the airway must be linked to a muscle sensitivity that is seen as bronchial hyper-reactivity.

Types of asthma

Types of asthma

Childhood onset—Usually atopic, tends to have pronounced variability and obvious precipitants.
Adult onset—Often more persistent, often few known precipitants except infection.
Occupational—Underdiagnosed, needs careful evaluation.
Nocturnal—Common in all types, relates to poor overall control and increased reactivity.
Cough-variant—May precede airflow obstruction, responds to treatment.
Exercise-induced—Common precipitant, may be the main problem in mild cases in children.

Asthma that develops during childhood usually varies considerably. Most young asthmatic patients have identifiable triggers that provoke wheezing although there is seldom one single extrinsic cause for all their attacks. This "extrinsic" asthma is often associated with other features of atopy such as rhinitis and eczema. When asthma starts in adult life the airflow obstruction is often more persistent and many exacerbations have no obvious stimuli other than respiratory tract infections. This pattern is often called "intrinsic" asthma. Immediate skin prick tests are less likely to be positive because of a lack of involvement of allergens or a loss of skin test positivity with age.

There are many patients who do not fit into these broad groups or who overlap the two types. There are other important types of asthma: one which presents with just a cough, and that related to occupational exposure.

Presentation with a cough is particularly common in children. Even in adults it should be considered as the cause of chronic unexplained cough. In some series of such cases asthma or a combination of rhinitis and asthma explained the cough in about half the patients who had been troubled by a cough with no obvious cause for more than two months.

Differential diagnosis

Differential diagnoses

Chronic bronchitis and emphysema—Difficult to differentiate in older smokers.

Large airway obstruction—Caused by foreign bodies and tumours, often misdiagnosed as asthma initially.

Pulmonary oedema—So-called "cardiac asthma", may include wheezing and may also occur at night.

The difficulty in breathing that is characteristic of asthma may be described as a constriction in the chest which suggests ischaemic cardiac pain. Nocturnal asthma that causes the patient to be woken from sleep by breathlessness may be confused with the paroxysmal nocturnal dyspnoea of heart failure.

After some years asthma, particularly when it is severe, may lose some or all of its reversibility. Chronic bronchitis and emphysema, usually caused by cigarette smoking, may show appreciable reversibility, which can make it quite difficult to be sure of the correct diagnosis in older patients with partially reversible obstruction. In practice, bronchodilators are given and corticosteroids used to establish the best airway function that can be achieved. The move to use inhaled corticosteroids for asthmatic patients who use their bronchodilators more than once a day may make management more difficult, because it is not just a question of establishing the best degree of reversibility possible with the bronchodilators. The role of regular inhaled corticosteroids in the treatment of chronic bronchitis and emphysema remains uncertain. Some studies have suggested that inhaled steroids slow the rate of decline of lung function with age, but more work is needed before they can be regarded as part of the routine treatment of chronic airflow obstruction. When there is reversibility to bronchodilators and any doubt whether the diagnosis might be asthma then inhaled corticosteroids should be part of the treatment.

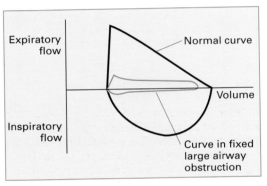

Flow volume curve.

Other causes of wheezing, such as obstruction of the large airways, occasionally produce problems in diagnosis. This may be the case with foreign bodies, particularly in children, or with tumours that gradually obstruct the trachea or main airways in adults. The noise produced is often a single pitched wheeze on inspiration and expiration rather than the multiple expiratory wheezes typical of asthma. Appropriate *x* rays and flow volume loops can show the site of obstruction. On spirometry the volume time curve may be a straight line.

Recording airflow obstruction

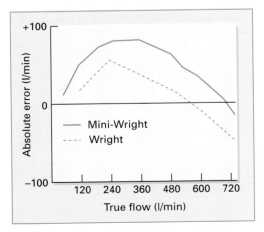

Errors in readings of Mini-Wright and Wright peak flow meters compared with flow from a pneumotachograph. Both over-read at lower flow rates and are non-linear.

"Mini" peak flow meters provide a cheap and reliable method of measuring airflow obstruction, and several are available on prescription. They may have errors that vary over the range of measurement but patients using the same peak flow meter over time can build up a pattern of their asthma which can be important in changing their treatment and planning management. The measurements add an objective element to subjective feelings of shortness of breath.

Although acute attacks of asthma occasionally have a sudden catastrophic onset they are more usually preceded by a gradual deterioration in control, which may not be noticed until it is quite advanced. An appreciable minority of patients are unaware of moderate changes in their airflow obstruction even when these occur acutely, and these patients are at particular risk of an acute exacerbation without warning. When such patients are identified they should be encouraged to take regular peak flow recordings and enter them on a diary card to permit them to see trends in peak flow measurements and react to exacerbations at an early stage before there is any change in their symptoms.

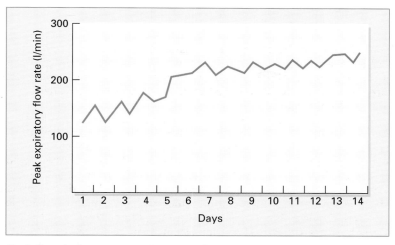

Peak flow during a two week course of oral corticosteroids in persistent asthma. The response plateaus at days 9–10.

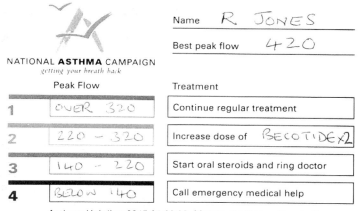

NATIONAL **ASTHMA** CAMPAIGN
getting your breath back

Name   R. JONES

Best peak flow   420

	Peak Flow	Treatment
1	OVER 320	Continue regular treatment
2	220 – 320	Increase dose of BECOTIDE×2
3	140 – 220	Start oral steroids and ring doctor
4	BELOW 140	Call emergency medical help

Asthma Helpline 0345 01 02 03, Monday to Friday, 9am to 9pm

Diagram of reactivity and trigger factors.

	Symptoms	Treatment
1	Asthma under control	Continue regular treatment
2	Getting a cold or waking with asthma at night	Increase dose of BECOTIDE × 2
3	Increasing breathlessness or poor response to	Start oral steroids and ring doctor
4	Severe attack	Call emergency medical help

Issued by   GUYS HOSPITAL   Date   MARCH 1994

National Asthma Campaign is a registered charity, number 802364

Details of the asthma credit card produced by the National Asthma Campaign as a brief reminder to patients.

"Mini" peak flow meters cost about £10 and have an important role in educating patients about their asthma. They should be used much more widely and be regarded as the equivalent in asthma of the regular urine or blood testing common among diabetic patients. It is not enough simply to give out a peak flow meter. Based on the home recordings, the doctor and the asthmatic patient can work together to develop plans with criteria that indicate the need for a change in treatment, a visit to the doctor, or emergency admission to hospital. This management plan should be written down for the patient and should be reviewed periodically. It has not been possible to show an effect on the control of asthma or hospital admission from the use of a peak flow meter alone, but a personal asthma management plan backed up by regular follow-up does improve control.

DIAGNOSTIC TESTING

Responsiveness to bronchodilators

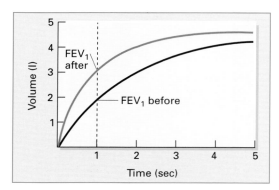

Spirometric response to treatment with a bronchodilator.

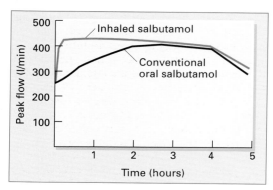

Effect of drugs on peak flow over time.

Responses to bronchodilators are easy to measure in the clinic or surgery. Reversibility is often used to establish the diagnosis of asthma or to find out which is the most effective bronchodilator. Reversibility is usually assessed by recording the best of three peak flow measurements, and then repeating the measurements 15–30 minutes after the patient has inhaled two or more doses of a β-agonist, salbutamol or terbutaline, from a metered dose inhaler or dry powder system. The method of inhalation should be supervised and the opportunity taken to correct the technique or change to a different inhalation device if necessary. The 95% confidence intervals for a change in peak flow rate on such repetitions are around 60 to 70 l/second. When forced expiratory volume in one second (FEV_1) is the measurement used, a change of 200 ml is outside the variability of the test. If a standard dose of a β-agonist does not produce a change, the peak flow can be measured again after either a larger dose of β–agonist or β-agonist combined with an anticholinergic agent, ipratropium or oxitropium bromide. These two agents are slower to act than β-agonists and their effect should be assessed 40–60 minutes after inhalation.

When there is severe obstruction and reversibility is limited, the application of strict reversibility criteria may be inappropriate. Any response may be worthwhile so attention should be paid to subjective responses and improvement of exercise tolerance together with results of other tests of respiratory function. Reversibility shown by other tests such as those of lung volumes or trapped gas volumes without changes in peak flow or FEV_1 are more likely to occur in patients with chronic bronchitis and emphysema than with asthma.

Decisions about treatment from such single dose studies should be backed up by further objective and subjective measurements during long term treatment. Responses to bronchodilators are not always consistent and, in some patients, changes after single doses in the laboratory may not predict the responses to the same drug over more prolonged periods.

Diurnal variation

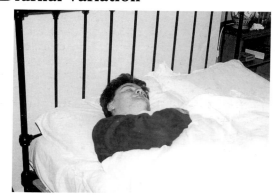

Lowest peak flow values occur in the early hours of the morning

A characteristic of asthma is a cyclical variation in the degree of airflow obstruction throughout the day. The lowest peak flow values occur in the early hours of the morning and the highest in the afternoon. To see the pattern a peak flow meter should be used at least twice and up to four times a day. Untreated asthmatic patients usually show a difference of at least 15% between mean morning and evening values. Many reasons have been suggested. The cause is still not clear and a combination of factors is probably involved.

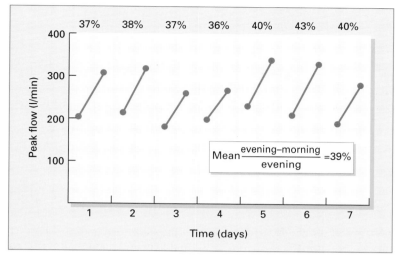

Diurnal variation in peak flow readings (%).

Documentation of diurnal variation by recording measurements from a peak flow meter shows typical diagnostic patterns in many patients. The timing of the measurements should be recorded, otherwise typical variations can be obscured by later readings at the weekend or on days away from work or school. In non-asthmatic subjects there is a small degree of diurnal variation with the same timing.

People with asthma commonly complain of waking at night. Large studies in the United Kingdom suggest that more than half of those with asthma have their sleep disturbed by an attack more than once a week. Deaths from asthma are also more likely to occur in the early hours of the morning.

Exercise testing

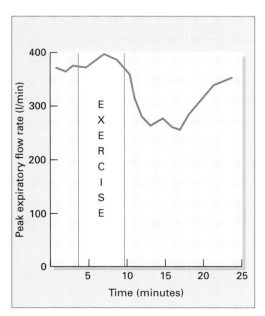

Exercise testing on a treadmill.

The provocation test most often used in the United Kingdom is a simple exercise test.

Exercise testing is a safe, simple procedure and may be useful when the diagnosis of asthma is in doubt. When baseline lung function is low, provocation testing is unnecessary for diagnosis as reversibility can be shown by bronchodilatation. Exercise testing and the recording of diurnal variations are used when the history suggests asthma but lung function is normal when the patient is seen. An exercise test may consist of baseline peak flow measurements, then six minutes of vigorous exercise such as running, followed by peak flow measurements for 20 minutes afterwards. The exercise is best done outside because breathing cold dry air intensifies the response. The characteristic asthmatic response is a fall in peak flow of more than 15% several minutes after the end of exercise. About 90% of asthmatic children will show a drop in peak flow in response to exercise. Once the peak flow rate has fallen by 15% the bronchoconstriction should be reversed by inhalation of a bronchodilator. Late reactions about six hours after challenge are unusual; unlike challenge with an allergen, patients do not need to be kept under observation for late responses after the initial response has been reversed. Such exercise tests are best avoided if the patient has ischaemic heart disease, but there is no reason why peak flow measurements should not be included during supervised exercise testing for coronary artery disease where this is appropriate.

The exercise test relies on changes in temperature and in the osmolality of the airway mucosa. Other challenge tests that rely on similar mechanisms include isocapnic hyperventilation; breathing cold, dry air; or osmotic challenge with nebulised distilled water or hypertonic saline. These are, however, laboratory-based procedures while the simple exercise test for asthma can be done at any clinic or surgery. Bronchodilators and sodium cromoglycate should be stopped at least six hours before the exercise test, and long-acting oral or inhaled bronchodilators should be stopped for at least 24 hours. Prolonged use of inhaled corticosteroids reduces responses to exercise but these are not usually stopped before testing because the effect takes days or weeks to wear off.

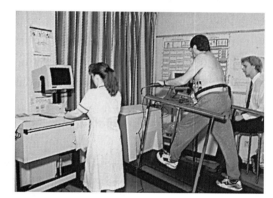

Decrease in peak expiratory flow rate in response to exercise.

Bronchial reactivity

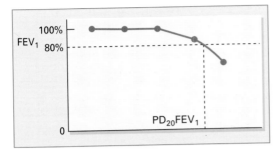

Log dose of histamine or methacholine.

Non-asthmatic patients do not develop bronchoconstriction on exercise; indeed, they usually show a small degree of bronchodilatation during the exercise itself. Other common forms of non-specific challenge to the airways are the inhalation of methacholine and histamine. These tests produce a range of responses usually defined as the dose of the challenging agent necessary to produce a drop in the FEV_1 of 20%. This is calculated by giving increasing doses until the FEV_1 drops below 80% of the baseline measurement, then drawing a line to connect the last two points above and below a 20% drop and taking the dose at the point on this line equivalent to a 20% drop in FEV_1. Nearly all patients with asthma show increased responsiveness, whereas patients with hay fever and not asthma form an intermediate group. This responsiveness of asthmatic patients has been associated with the underlying inflammation in the airway wall.

The degree of responsiveness is associated with the severity of the airways disease. It can be reduced by strict avoidance of known allergens or by the use of drugs such as corticosteroids to reduce the inflammation in the wall of the airway. Use of a bronchodilator is followed by a temporary reduction while the mechanisms of smooth muscle contraction are blocked. Bronchial reactivity is an important epidemiological and research tool. In clinical practice it has little place except with difficult diagnostic problems such as persistent cough.

Specific airway challenge

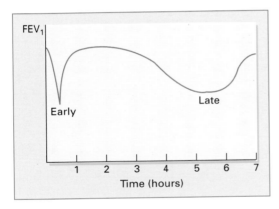

Challenge with agents to which a patient is thought to be sensitive must be done with caution. The initial dose should be low and, even so, reactions may be unpredictable. Early narrowing of the airway by contraction of smooth muscle occurs within the first 30 minutes and there is often a "late response" 4–8 hours later. The late response may be followed by poorer control of the asthma and greater diurnal variation for days or weeks afterwards. The late response is thought to be associated with release of mediators and attraction of inflammatory cells to the airways. It has been used in drug development as a more suitable model for clinical asthma than the brief early response.

Challenges with specific allergens are used mostly for the investigation of occupational asthma but they should be restricted to experienced laboratories and patients should be supervised for at least eight hours after challenge.

Skin tests

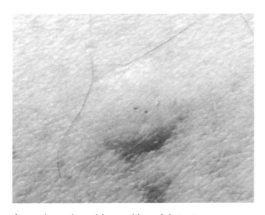

A weal produced by a skin prick test.

In skin prick tests a small amount of the test substance is introduced into the superficial layers of the epidermis on the tip of a small needle. The tests are painless. Most young asthmatics show a range of positive responses to common allergens such as house dust mite, pollens, and animal dander. A weal that develops 15 minutes after a skin prick test suggests the presence of specific IgE antibody, and the results correlate well with those of in vitro tests for IgE such as the radioallergosorbent test (RAST), which is more expensive.

Positive skin tests do not establish a diagnosis of asthma or the importance of the specific allergens used. They show only the tendency to produce IgE to common allergens—atopy. More than 20% of the population have positive skin tests, but less than a half of these will develop asthma. The prevalence and strength of positive skin tests declines with age.

The importance of allergic factors in asthma is best ascertained from a careful clinical history, taking into account seasonal factors and trials of avoidance of allergens. Suspicions can be confirmed by skin tests or, less often, by specific inhalation challenge.

Although positive skin tests do not incriminate the allergen as a cause of the patient's asthma it would be rare for an inhalant to be important in asthma with a negative skin test. The results do, however, rely on the quality of the agents used in testing and will be negative if antihistamines are being taken. Corticosteroids have no appreciable effect on immediate skin prick tests.

CLINICAL COURSE

Growing out of asthma

Asthma: things to avoid
• Known allergens
• Active and passive cigarette smoking
• Areas of high pollution (particularly exercise at times of high air pollution)
• β-Blockers
• Aspirin and non-steroidal anti-inflammatory drugs.

Parents of asthmatic children are usually concerned about whether their child will "grow out of" asthma. Most wheezy children improve during their teens but the outlook depends to some extent on the severity of their early disease.

Over half the children whose wheezing is infrequent will be free of symptoms by the time they are 21, but of those with frequent, troublesome wheezing only 20% will be symptom free at 21, although 20% will be substantially better. In 15% of patients, the asthma becomes more troublesome in early adult years than it was in childhood. Even if there is prolonged remission lasting several years symptoms may return later. After months free of symptoms the airway epithelium may still be inflamed and airway reactivity may remain abnormally high. This suggests that the underlying tendency to be asthmatic remains and a third of the children who have a year's remission will get further symptoms years later.

Asthma is less likely to go into remission in patients with a strong family history of atopy or a personal history of other atopic conditions, low respiratory function, onset after the age of 29, and frequent attacks. More boys than girls are affected by asthma but the girls do less well during adolescence and by adulthood the sex ratio is equal. Most of those who do grow out of asthma are left with no residual effects other than the risk of recrudescence. Chest deformities are uncommon and only occur when there is severe, intractable disease.

Although puberty may be delayed, the final adult height of children with asthma is usually normal unless they have received long term treatment with systemic or high-dose inhaled corticosteroids.

Prognosis in adults

Types of drug used in asthma
For relief
• Inhaled β-agonists
• Inhaled anticholinergics
Regular bronchodilators
• Theophyllines
• Oral β-agonists
• Long acting β-agonists
For prophylaxis
• Inhaled corticosteroids
• Sodium cromoglycate
• Nedocromil sodium

Asthma in adults often shows less spontaneous variation than it does in children. Wheezing is more persistent and there is less association with obvious precipitating factors other than infections. The chances of a sustained remission are also lower than in children. Smokers with increased bronchial reactivity are particularly at risk of developing chronic airflow obstruction and it is vital that asthmatic patients do not smoke. When there are known precipitating agents which can be avoided such as animals or occupational factors then removal of these will reduce bronchial reactivity. The avoidance of contact with known allergens can reduce responses to non-specific agents including cigarette smoke, cold air, and dust, and lead to an improvement in both the control and the progress of the asthma.

The reversibility of airways obstruction in asthma is not always maintained throughout life. Those with more severe asthma are most likely to go on to develop irreversible airflow obstruction. It is likely that this progression to irreversibility is related to persistent inflammation of the wall of the airway, which leads to permanent damage. Suitable prolonged prophylaxis reduces the inflammation and most chest physicians act on the belief that this will reduce the likelihood of long term damage and eventual irreversibility. There are few prolonged studies to prove or disprove this contention but the benefits of anti-inflammatory prophylaxis are well established in the short term and it seems prudent to follow this practice.

Individual management plan

Preventer
1 Take the Pulmicort (brown) once in morning and once at night *every* day.
2 If you get a cold or peak flow drops below 300 l/min take two doses morning and night.
Reliever
1 Take the Ventolin (blue) two puffs when you need it.
2 If you need it more than five times a day get an appointment.
Action
1 Peak flow less than 250 l/min start prednisolone six tablets a day and get an appointment within 48 hours.
2 Peak flow less than 200 l/min and wheezy, take six prednisolone tablets, four puffs Ventolin, and ring surgery or go to Casualty.

Educating patients about their asthma and the use of treatment is an integral part of management. Patients forget much of what they are told in consultations and information should be backed up by written instructions. It is often helpful to produce these in a handwritten form for each patient. Standard written information from asthma societies and other sources can be used as a backup but a personal plan is preferable. Patients are often confused about the differences between regular prophylaxis, such as inhaled corticosteroids or sodium cromoglycate, and the quickly effective inhaled bronchodilators used to treat acute attacks. Regular use of a mini peak flow meter allows the patient to participate more effectively in the understanding and treatment of the disease. Even with this information, though, many patients do not adhere to their prescribed regimen. Only half of all asthmatic patients achieve 75% compliance with their prescribed treatment. This is true for all chronic conditions and shows the need for regular reinforcement, matching the information to the patients, and for further work in the area of education and compliance.

Genetic factors and clinical course

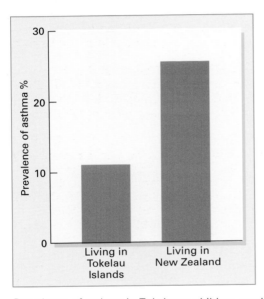

Prevalence of asthma in Tokelauan children aged 0–14 years still in the Tokelau Islands or resettled in New Zealand. Asthma, rhinitis, and eczema were all more prevalent in islanders who had been resettled in New Zealand after a hurricane. Environmental factors have an effect as well as genetic predisposition.

There is a familial element in asthma. Atopic subjects are at risk of asthma and rhinitis; they can be identified by positive immediate skin prick tests to common allergens. It has been suggested that there is a distinct gene for atopy on chromosome 11q but that transmission occurs only through the maternal line. Other studies have not confirmed such a close relationship to the gene locus on 11q. It is likely that the pattern of inheritance may be more complicated than a single gene pattern and that the different patterns found so far may depend on the choice of the families selected in the study.

The development of asthma depends on environmental factors acting with a genetic predisposition. The movement of racial groups with a low prevalence of asthma from an isolated rural environment to an urban area increases the prevalence in that group, possibly because of their increased exposure to allergens such as house dust mites and fungal spores or to infectious agents, pollution, and dietary changes.

The chance of a person developing asthma by the age of 50 years is increased 10 times if there is a first degree relative with asthma. The risk is greater the more severe the relative's asthma. It has been suggested that breast feeding may reduce the risk of a child developing atopic conditions such as asthma because it restricts the exposure to ingested foreign protein in the first few months of life. Conflicting studies have been published and it may require considerable dietary restriction by the mother to avoid passing antigen on to the child during this vulnerable period.

Maternal smoking in pregnancy increases the risk of childhood asthma, and exposure during the first few years of life is also detrimental. Studies of paternal smoking have produced less certain trends in the same direction.

Deaths from asthma

Asthmatic patients who have severe attacks attacks have reduced responses to hypoxia and to increased respiratory load. The lower sensitivity may allow them to deteriorate further before seeking help. They are a vulnerable group and need to be monitored carefully.

Since the sharp temporary increase in mortality from asthma seen in some countries during the early 1960s there has been concern about the role of treatment in such deaths. The deaths in the 1960s have been attributed to cardiac stimulation caused by overuse of inhaled isoprenaline, or to excessive reliance on its usual efficacy after delay in using appropriate alternative treatment when symptoms worsened. Isoprenaline as a bronchodilator has been superseded by safer β_2–stimulants.

After the peak in the 1960s the number of deaths from asthma in the United Kingdom stabilised. In the late 1980s there was a suggestion of a gradual rise in deaths to about 2000/year. The figures are most reliable for the 5–34 year age group and the most recent figures suggest that there may have been a slight fall in mortality.

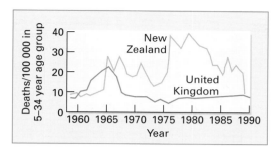

Asthma mortality 1958–1990 in the United Kingdom and New Zealand. Both rose in the 1960s, and in New Zealand there was a further rise in the late 1970s which has now resolved.

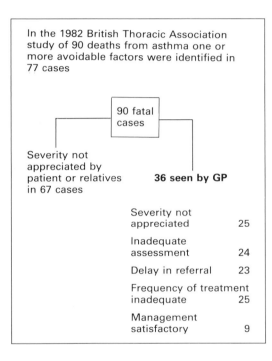

In the 1982 British Thoracic Association study of 90 deaths from asthma one or more avoidable factors were identified in 77 cases

90 fatal cases

Severity not appreciated by patient or relatives in 67 cases

36 seen by GP

Severity not appreciated	25
Inadequate assessment	24
Delay in referral	23
Frequency of treatment inadequate	25
Management satisfactory	9

Morbidity

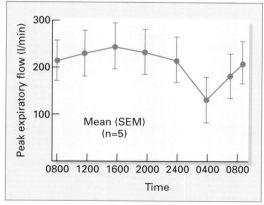

Peak flow measurements can be used to confirm the diagnosis of nocturnal asthma. Decreases in the early hours are associated with disturbed sleep and daytime tiredness.

In the 1980s mortality from asthma in New Zealand rose appreciably. Once again the reasons are uncertain and have aroused controversy. The increase in deaths in New Zealand has been reversed and has not been mirrored elsewhere. The combination of methylxanthines and β_2–stimulants, and the use of home nebulisers, were blamed but neither provided a satisfactory explanation for the problems. In New Zealand fenoterol was a popular β_2–agonist and it has been linked to the increase in mortality because it is claimed that it has more cardiac stimulating effects than other β_2–agonists and that it was marketed in a higher strength dose for dose than in the United Kingdom. An alternative suggestion was that it was used in more severe cases but an attempt to explore this hypothesis by retrospective case matching did not support the explanation. These doubts fuelled worries about the possibility that β–agonists might have the potential to worsen control of asthma and increase morbidity and even mortality.

Investigation of the circumstances surrounding individual deaths generally finds evidence of undertreatment rather than excessive medication in such deaths. Both doctors and patients underestimate the severity of attacks, and the most important factor may be an apparent reluctance to take oral corticosteroids for severe asthmatic episodes and to adjust treatment early during periods of deterioration. Nevertheless, about a quarter of deaths occur less than an hour after the start of an exacerbation, and patients who have such rapid deterioration are particularly vulnerable. If patients have deteriorated swiftly in the past they should have suitable treatment, such as steroids and nebulised and injectable bronchodilators, readily available. They and their relatives must be confident in the use of their emergency treatment and know how to obtain further help immediately.

Several centres have adopted the policy recommended in Edinburgh of maintaining a self admission service for selected asthmatic patients. This avoids delay in admitting patients to hospital and is a logical development of involving patients in the management of their own disease.

Some studies have shown that patients are particularly at risk after they have been discharged from intensive care or high dependency units to ordinary wards and after discharge from hospital. Problems often occur in the early hours of the morning, at the nadir of the diurnal cycle, and may be related to premature tailing off of the initial intensive treatment because the measurements during the day have been satisfactory. Adequate supervision and treatment must be maintained throughout these periods.

Assessment and management in hospital have also been criticised. Asthma has proved to be a popular subject for audit according to the consensus guidelines of the British Thoracic Society. Many studies have shown that initial assessment and treatment are satisfactory but that there are weaknesses in the exploration of reasons for an attack, establishment of suitable control before discharge, and follow up arrangements. Every admission should be regarded as a failure of routine management. Quality of treatment, readmission rates and asthma control are improved when the inpatient care is supervised by those with an interest in thoracic medicine.

Asthma causes considerable morbidity with persistent symptoms and loss of time from work and school. Sleep is disturbed by asthma more than once a week in over half the patients and this leads to poorer daytime performance. There has been a shift in the general approach to management aiming to produce freedom from symptoms rather than a tolerable existence free of disabling attacks. This is a major message in the 1993 guidelines from the British Thoracic Society. It requires a more aggressive approach early in the course of the disease with regular anti-inflammatory drugs and will, it is hoped, lead to a reduction in morbidity from exacerbations of asthma and long term damage.

PRECIPITATING FACTORS

Bronchial reactivity

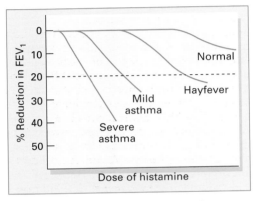

Bronchial reactivity is increased in asthma, particularly in more severe disease.

The concept of bronchial reactivity of the airway to specific and non-specific stimuli is discussed in chapter 2.

The underlying cause of increased bronchial reactivity is uncertain. The sustained reactivity found in asthmatic patients has been attributed to imbalance of autonomic control or other non-adrenergic, non-cholinergic plexuses, abnormal immunological and cellular responses, increased permeability of the epithelium, and intrinsic differences in the action of smooth muscle or its hypertrophy.

Airways in asthmatic patients are usually sensitive to non-specific stimuli such as dust and smoke. Laughing or coughing may provoke wheezing. Specific responses to agents such as pollen may lead to increased non-specific reactivity and symptoms of asthma for days or even weeks. Upper respiratory viral infections may lead to similar changes and may increase reactivity in non-asthmatic subjects. Challenge to airways by specific allergens may induce late responses 6–10 hours after exposure. Such late responses may mimic more closely the inflammatory changes caused by asthma that occur spontaneously. They lead to a subsequent rise in non-specific airway reactivity.

Exercise

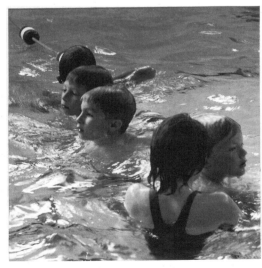

Premedication with a β_2-stimulant or sodium cromoglycate usually allows asthmatic children to participate in sports.

Vigorous exercise produces narrowing of the airways in most asthmatic patients and, as described in the second chapter, can be used as a simple diagnostic test. Asthma during or after exercise is most likely to be a practical problem in children, where it may interfere with games at school. The type of exercise influences the response; most asthmatic patients find that swimming in warm indoor pools is the activity that is least likely to induce an attack. This clinical observation has been explained by studies showing the importance of cooling and drying of the airways during hyperventilation and exercise. The effect of exercise can be mimicked by breathing cold, dry air, whereas breathing warm, humid air—as in indoor swimming pools—prevents the asthmatic response. In some patients, however, this picture is confused, because they are sensitive to the chemical agents used in swimming pools.

The best protection against exercise–induced asthma is inhalation of a β_2–stimulant beforehand. Sodium cromoglycate and nedocromil sodium are also usually effective, and such treatment will normally allow a child to take part in games at school. It may be necessary to explain to the teachers the use of drugs and the objectives of the treatment. Exercise itself is unlikely to have any major beneficial effect on asthma, but general fitness and activity should be encouraged. A fit person can do a given task with less overall ventilation than an unfit one, and hence less chance of exercise–induced asthma. Asthma is quite compatible with a successful sporting career as a number of athletes have testified in manufacturers' advertisements, and the common inhaled asthma drugs are allowed in the regulations of most sporting bodies. The exceptions are fenoterol and Intal Compound (which includes isoprenaline).

A second bout of exercise within an hour or so of the first is often less troublesome, a phenomenon known as refractoriness. The general benefits of warming up before exercise may therefore be increased for asthmatic athletes. Late asthmatic responses 4–6 hours after exposure are common after exposure to allergens, but they are rare and not troublesome after exercise.

> Asthmatic athletes should always warm up before exercise.

House dust mites

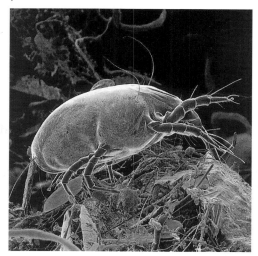

Scanning electron micrograph of a house dust mite.

The house dust mite, *Dermatophagoides pteronyssinus*, provides the material for the commonest positive skin prick test in the United Kingdom. The main allergen is found in the mites' faecal pellets. The mites live off human skin scales; are widely distributed in bedding, furniture, carpets, and soft toys; and thrive best in warm, damp conditions. The expectation of a warm environment at home has increased the exposure of children to allergens and is likely to be an important element in the increased prevalence of asthma.

If patients move into environments that are free of house dust mites their symptoms improve. This can be achieved in the mountains of Switzerland or, nearer to home but less picturesque, in specially cleaned hospital wards without soft furnishings. It is more difficult to reduce the numbers of mites sufficiently in the home. Regular cleaning of bedrooms and avoiding materials that are particularly likely to collect dust are sensible measures to keep down the antigenic load. More rigorous mite reduction has been attempted with mattress covers that are impermeable to mites, fine filters on vacuum cleaners, acaricides, or even applications of liquid nitrogen to mattresses. A concerted effort can reduce the number of mites low enough to improve control of asthma, but none of these interventions has a routine role. Desensitisation to house dust mites may be of some use in children.

Pollens and spores

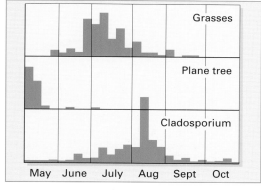

Seasonal variations in allergens.

Seasonal asthma, often together with rhinitis and conjunctivitis, is most usually associated with grass pollens, which are most common during June and July. Less common in the United Kingdom is precipitation of asthma by tree pollens, many of which are produced between February and May, and mould spores from *Cladosporium* and *Alternaria* which abound in July and August. Complete avoidance of such widespread pollens is impractical.

The effectiveness of hyposensitisation is debatable. It is generally unnecessary because inhaled drugs usually produce adequate control and are simple to use. The strong placebo effect, allergic reactions to hyposensitisation, and the occasional mortality must also be taken into account in assessing its value.

Allergic bronchopulmonary aspergillosis

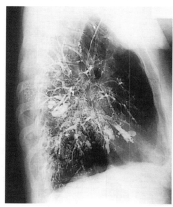

Bronchiectasis in a case of allergic bronchopulmonary aspergillosis.

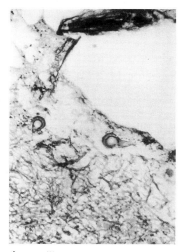

Aspergillus fumigatus hyphae and conidiophores (fruiting heads).

Some asthmatic patients develop a sensitivity to the spores of *Aspergillus fumigatus*, which is a common fungus particularly partial to rotting vegetation. Allergic bronchopulmonary aspergillosis is associated with eosinophilia in blood and sputum, rubbery brownish plugs of mucus containing fungal hyphae, and proximal bronchiectasis. Areas of consolidation and collapse may be visible in the chest *x* ray film, and each episode can lead to further bronchiectatic damage. The aspergillus skin test will be positive and specific IgE will be found in the blood. Individual episodes settle after treatment with corticosteroids but if they are frequent and bronchiectasis is developing then long term oral corticosteroids may be appropriate. Antifungal imidazoles such as itraconazole may also reduce the frequency of attacks.

Precipitating factors

Pets

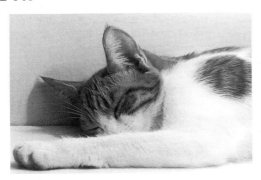

The parents of asthmatic children often worry about household pets. Cats cause the greatest problem, with allergens in saliva, urine, and dander, but most domestic animals can trigger asthma on occasions. Patients who have major problems with their asthma should be advised not to acquire any new pets. When children are born into a family with a strong history of atopy then furry and hairy pets are best avoided. Pets already in residence should be kept out of bedrooms and off soft furnishings. If the animal seems to be a cause of serious symptoms then a trial separation should be organised. Animal allergens remain in the house long after the pet is removed so the pet should move out for a month or two; alternatively the patient could move out for a week or two. Unjustified removal of favourite pets without good reason may, however, provoke more serious problems from emotional upset.

Occupational asthma

Some causes of occupational asthma

Chemicals	Isocyanates
	Platinum salts
	Epoxy resins
	Aluminium
	Hair sprays
	Azodicarbonamide
	(plastic blowing)
Vegetable sources	Wood dusts
	Grains
	Coffee beans
	Colophony (solders)
	Cotton, flax, hemp dust
	Castor bean dust
Enzymes	Trypsin
	Bacillus subtilis
Animals	Laboratory rodents
	Larger mammals
	Shellfish
	Locusts
	Grain weevil, mites
Drug manufacture	Penicillins
	Piperazine
	Salbutamol
	Cimetidine
	Ispaghula
	Ipecacuanha

The importance of occupational asthma is being increasingly recognised. Some estimates suggest that over 5% of cases of adult asthma have an occupational origin and over 200 precipitating agents have been reported. Asthmatic patients choosing a career should avoid occupations where they are likely to be exposed to large quantities of non-specific stimuli such as dust and cold air.

Occupational asthma is officially recognised as an industrial disease and subject to compensation. It is defined as "asthma which develops after a variable period of symptomless exposure to a sensitising agent at work." Fourteen agents are currently recognised for compensation and this list is kept under regular review. Agents such as proteolytic enzymes and laboratory animals are particularly likely to produce problems in atopic subjects, whereas isocyanate asthma is not related to atopic status. In some studies potent agents such as platinum salts have produced asthma in up to half of those who are exposed to them.

Increased bronchial reactivity provoked by occupational agents may persist long after removal from exposure. Regular peak flow recordings are once again an important diagnostic tool and usually show a distinct relation to time at work, but the relationship may not be obvious because the timing of the responses is variable. Reactions may occur soon after arriving at work, be delayed until later in the day, or come on slowly over several days. In some cases a weekend away from work may not be long enough for lung function to return to normal and absence for a week or two may be necessary. Initial investigations include exploration of potential agents at work and recording peak flow patterns 2 or 4 hourly at and away from work. Further investigation may require specific challenge testing in an experienced laboratory.

The first approach to management should be to try to adjust the conditions at work which produced the sensitisation. If this is not possible the patient may be able to continue working with a mask to provide filtered air. If these measures fail and simple inhaled treatment is inadequate then a change of job will be necessary. It is advisable to try to obtain, with the patient's consent, the cooperation of any occupational health staff in the firm.

Food allergy

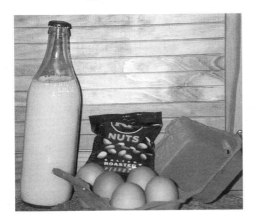

Food allergy causes eczema and gastrointestinal symptoms more often than asthma, but some striking cases do occur. Exclusion diets have generally been disappointing in asthma, and immediate skin prick tests and radioallergosorbent tests are less useful than for inhaled allergens. Most serious cases of asthma induced by food intolerance are evident from a carefully taken history, so elaborate diets are not warranted. When there is doubt, suspicions can be confirmed by excluding the agent from the diet or by controlled exposure.

Intolerance to food does not always indicate an allergic mechanism. Reactions may be related to pharmacological mediators such as histamine or tyramine in the food. They may be produced by food additives such as the yellow dye tartrazine, which is added to a wide range of foods and medications. When there is a specific allergy to foodstuffs, the most likely to be implicated are milk, eggs, nuts, and wheat.

Drug-induced asthma

Two main groups of drugs are responsible for most cases of drug induced asthma: β-blocking agents and prostaglandin sythetase inhibitors such as aspirin. β-blocking agents usually induce bronchoconstriction when given to asthmatic patients and this may happen even when they are given in eye drops. Relatively selective β-blockers such as atenolol and metoprolol are less likely to cause severe irreversible asthma, but the whole group of β-blocking drugs should be avoided in patients who already have asthma. For hypertension, diuretics, angiotensin converting enzyme inhibitors, or calcium antagonists are suitable alternatives. Calcium antagonists can also be used for angina and may even be beneficial in partially blocking exercise–induced asthma. When asthma is produced by β–blockade, large doses of β–stimulants are necessary to reverse it, particularly with less selective β–blockers. Fortunately, cardiac side effects of treatment with β–stimulants are not a problem because they are also inhibited by the β–blockade.

Salicylates provoke severe narrowing of the airways in a small group of adults with asthma. Once such a reaction has been noted these patients should avoid contact with aspirin or non-steroidal anti-inflammatory agents which usually produce the same effects. The mechanism is probably related to changes in arachidonic acid metabolism. Milder salicylate sensitivity can be shown more often on routine testing, particularly in adults with asthma and nasal polyps.

Ibuprofen is available without prescription and has the same effects. Patients are often unaware of the presence of salicylate in common compound preparations and cold cures. When salicylate sensitivity is suspected the patient should be asked to check carefully the contents of any such medication they take. When salicylate reactions occur it may be possible to induce tolerance by carefully building up from small oral doses. This should be done only in experienced units.

Occasionally drugs used to treat asthma can themselves be responsible for provoking bronchoconstriction. Such paradoxical effects have been described with aminophylline, ipratropium bromide, sodium cromoglycate, β-agonists in infants, and propellants or contaminants from the valve apparatus in metered dose inhalers.

Hypotonic solutions are a potent cause of bronchoconstriction in people with asthma, and nebuliser solutions must always be made up with normal saline rather than water. Preservatives in nebuliser solutions have also produced narrowing of the airways.

Drugs that cause drug-induced asthma

- β-blockers (including eye drops)
- Aspirin
- Non-steroidal anti-inflammatory drugs
- Inhaled asthma drugs
- Nebuliser solutions, hypotonic or with preservatives
- Angiotensin converting enzyme inhibitors

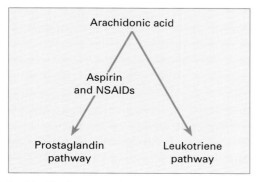

Aspirin blocks prostaglandin synthetase activity and sends arachidonic acid metabolism down the leukotriene pathway. This is likely to be the basis of aspirin-induced asthma.

Emotional factors

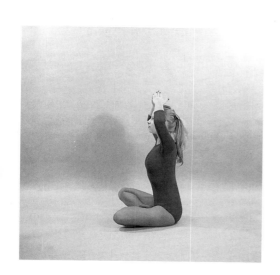

Psychological factors can play an important part in asthma. On their own they do not produce asthma in subjects without an underlying susceptibility, but in the laboratory emotional factors and expectation can influence both the bronchoconstrictor responses to various specific and non-specific stimuli and the bronchodilator responses to treatment. Stress and emotional disturbance are factors that must be taken into account in the overall management of asthmatic patients. In children the position is complicated by the emotional responses of their parents. Emotional problems are more likely to occur when control of asthma is poor, and these problems are best managed by increasing the confidence of patients and relatives with adequate explanation and control of the asthma. It is particularly important that patients know exactly what to do during an acute exacerbation. More specific measures such as relaxation, yoga, hypnotherapy, and acupuncture have been investigated. Some trials have shown beneficial effects and some patients obtain considerable help from relaxation treatment. If conventional medicines are neglected when alternative approaches are adopted, however, it can be dangerous.

Asthma associated with emotional outbursts such as laughing and crying may be related to the response of the hyper–reactive airways to deep inspirations or to inhalation of cold, dry air rather than to the emotion itself.

Manipulative patients may, of course, use a disease such as asthma for their own purposes just as they might use any other chronic disease.

Pollution

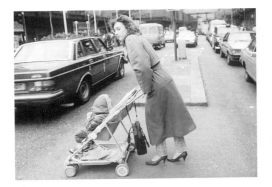

Personal air pollution with cigarette smoke worsens asthma; both active and passive smoking provoke narrowing of the airways.

There has been increased interest in environmental pollution lately. Though the inner city smogs of the 1950s and earlier disappeared after the introduction of the *Clean Air Act*, high levels of ozone, sulphur dioxide, oxides of nitrogen, and particulate matter develop in certain areas and in particular climatic conditions. Combinations of high temperature, humidity, and heavy traffic can cause levels above the WHO recommended guidelines. Asthmatics should be aware of measures of air quality, and whenever possible they should keep away from areas of high pollution particularly when exercising.

Climatic conditions such as the pressure and humidity associated with thunderstorms can provoke asthma. The conditions may increase the concentrations of fungal and pollen spores at ground level as they are brought down from higher levels of the atmosphere. The spores rupture to produce particles of respirable size.

Levels of nitrogen dioxide found in the home may increase airway responses to common allergens such as house dust mite.

Asthma and pregnancy

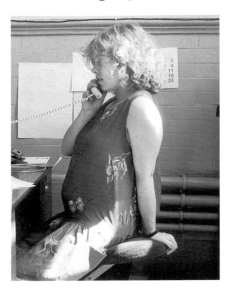

The control of asthma during pregnancy can change but the effect is variable. About a third of patients improve, a third worsen, and a third continue unchanged. The effect may vary among pregnancies in the same woman. Breathlessness may be more pronounced in late pregnancy as the diaphragmatic movement is limited even without any change in airflow obstruction.

There is a natural anxiety about the use of drugs during pregnancy. Fortunately the usual asthma treatments of inhaled β-antagonists, and inhaled and oral corticosteroids have been shown to be safe. Asthma control and supervision should be improved during pregnancy to reduce the likelihood of an acute exacerbation. Acute attacks should be treated vigorously in the normal way. Severe asthma and hypoxia rather than asthma treatments are the potential danger during pregnancy.

ACUTE ASTHMA: GENERAL MANAGEMENT

Assessment of severity

The speed of onset of acute attacks varies. Some severe episodes come on over a period of minutes with no warning, although more often there is a background of deterioration over days or weeks. This period during which control of the asthma deteriorates tends to be longer in older patients. A good early guide to developing problems is the need to use bronchodilator inhalers more often than usual, or finding that they are less effective. Deterioration in control can also be detected by regular monitoring of peak flow at home; a drop in the peak flow, or an increase in the diurnal variation of peak flow, provides evidence of instability. Detecting these changes allows a change of treatment while the decline is slow and before severe problems arise. All asthmatic patients should be aware of what to do if they fail to get relief from their usual treatment. A written action plan should be available for patients and relatives, which should include trigger levels of peak flow or symptoms which require changes in treatment or consultation for further advice.

Features of severe asthma

- Unable to speak a sentence in one breath
- Respiratory rate >25/minute
- Pulse rate >110/minute
- Peak flow rate <50% best known or predicted value

The most common symptom is breathlessness and there is more likely to be difficulty in inspiration than in expiration. A few patients have a poor appreciation of changes in the degree of their airflow obstruction and will complain of few symptoms until they have developed moderately severe asthma. They are at particular risk during acute attacks and are a group in which regular peak flow monitoring is particularly important.

Caution:
Patients with severe or life threatening attacks may not be distressed and may not have all these abnormalities.

As the severity of the asthma increases the breathlessness begins to interfere with simple functions. Exercise is limited and later eating and drinking are difficult. In severe attacks it will be difficult for the patient to speak in full sentences without gasping for breath between words. A knowledge of the pattern of previous attacks is important as the progress is often broadly similar in subsequent episodes. Patients must be taught to seek help early rather than late in an acute exacerbation; it is easier to step in and prevent deterioration into severe asthma rather than treat a full–blown attack. Patients and their families should all be confident about the management of exacerbations, both of their immediate treatment and the ways to get further help and hospital admission. These should all be discussed before the first acute attack of asthma.

Features of very severe, life threatening asthma

- Silent chest
- Cyanosis
- Poor respiratory effort
- Bradycardia or hypotension
- Exhaustion, confusion, or coma
- Peak flow rate <33% best known or predicted value
- Normal or high carbon dioxide tension (>5 kPa, 36 mm Hg)
- Severe hypoxia despite oxygen (<8 kPa, 60 mm Hg)
- Low pH

Acute asthma: general management

Examination

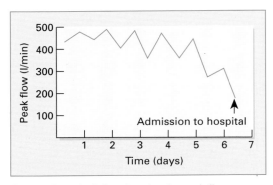

Graph of gradual deterioration in peak flow.

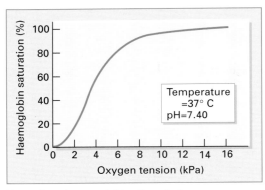

Normal oxyhaemoglobin dissociation curve.

Inability to speak will be obvious when taking the history. Respiratory rate is a useful sign and should be counted accurately; a rate of 25/minute or above is a sign of severity. Hypoxia severe enough to cause confusion occurs only in severe asthma and means that admission to hospital and supplemental oxygen are needed urgently. The pulse rate is also a useful guide to severity: a tachycardia over 110 beats/minute is found in severe episodes although this sign may be less reliable in the elderly when pulse rates tend to remain low. In very severe attacks bradycardia may occur. Pulsus paradoxus (a drop in systolic pressure of more than 10 mm Hg on inspiration) is not always present, even in severe asthma. A drop of over 20 mmHg is a sign of severe asthma, and changes correlate well with progress and can be one way to monitor the effects of treatment. Any evidence of circulatory embarrassment such as hypotension is an indication for admission to hospital.

Examination of the chest itself shows a fast respiratory rate, overinflation, and wheezing. In very severe acute asthma airflow may be too little for an audible wheeze, so a quiet chest during an acute attack is worrying rather than reassuring. It may also indicate a pneumothorax. Although pneumothoraces are not common in acute asthma they are difficult to diagnose clinically, and a chest x ray film must be taken if there is any doubt.

In severe attacks the peak flow rate may be unrecordable. Peak flow or FEV_1 should be monitored throughout the attack and during recovery as they are reliable, simple guides to the effectiveness of treatment. Peak flow values are easier to interpret if the patient's usual or best readings are known.

An initial measurement of blood gases should be done in patients with asthma severe enough to warrant admission to hospital. Great care should be taken with blood gas measurements because some asthmatic patients who have had bad experiences of arterial puncture may delay attendance at hospital because of the memories of pain. In patients with mild attacks a pulse oximeter should be used in the accident and emergency department. If saturation is 95% or above while breathing air and the patient does not have signs of severe asthma then blood gas measurement can be omitted. In more severe cases oxygen saturation by pulse oximeter can be used to assess progress after the first arterial gas measurement provided the initial carbon dioxide tension was not raised and there is no sign of appreciable deterioration.

Some hypoxia is usual and responds to supplemental oxygen. An arterial oxygen tension of less than 8kPa on air is a mark of severity. As long as the patient does not have chronic bronchitis and emphysema there is no need to limit the concentration of supplemental oxygen. The arterial carbon dioxide tension is usually low in acute asthma; occasionally it is high on admission, but it quickly responds to treatment with a bronchodilator, particularly in children. Hypercapnia is, however, an alarming feature of acute asthma and failure either to reduce carbon dioxide retention during the first hour or to prevent its development during treatment is an indication that mechanical ventilation must be considered. The final decision on this depends on the overall clinical state of the patient rather than on the blood gas measurement alone.

Where to treat acute asthma

Most of the people who die of acute asthma do so because the severity of the attack was underestimated.

An acute attack of asthma is frightening; conceivably transfer to hospital may exacerbate symptoms by producing anxiety, and reassurance that treatment is available to relieve the attack is an important part of the management. It is not possible to lay down strict criteria for admission to hospital. The features of severity discussed above should, however, be assessed. Most of the dangers of acute asthma come from a failure to appreciate the severity of an attack and the absence of suitable supervision and treatment to follow up the initial response. Immediate improvement after the first nebuliser treatment may provide false reassurance, being followed quickly by the return of severe asthma, so continued observation is essential.

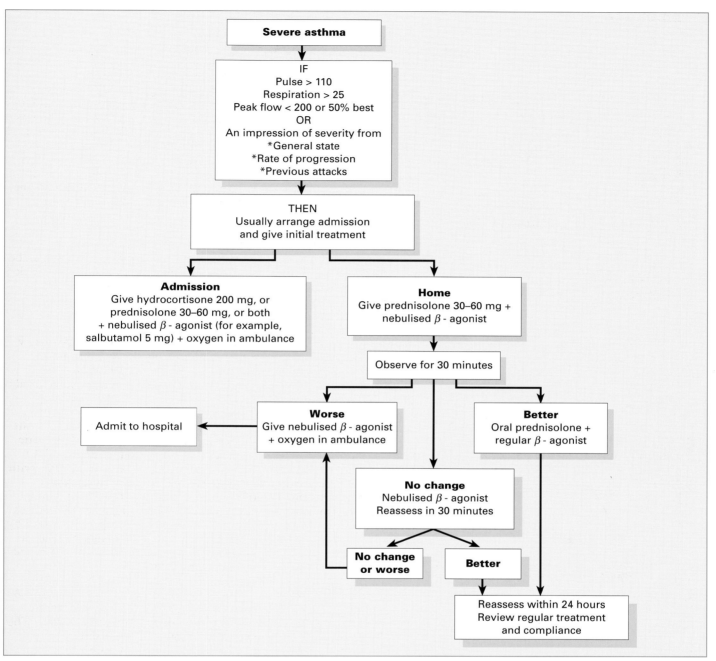

Treatment of adult acute severe asthma in general practice.

It may be obvious on first seeing the patient that supplemental oxygen and hospital treatment are necessary. Treatment should be started while this is arranged. In less severe attacks initial treatment should be given and, if the response is inadequate, hospital admission should be arranged. If the initial response is adequate it may be possible to manage the patient at home if supervision is available. The primary treatment should then be followed up, usually by adequate bronchodilation and corticosteroids, and the response should be assessed by measurements of peak flow.

Most deaths from asthma occur when the patient or doctor has failed to appreciate the severity of the attack. When there is any doubt it is safer to opt for vigorous treatment and admission to hospital. When treatment is given at home, the patient's condition must be assessed regularly and often until the exacerbation has settled. The reason for the acute exacerbation must then be sought.

TREATMENT OF ACUTE ASTHMA

Introduction

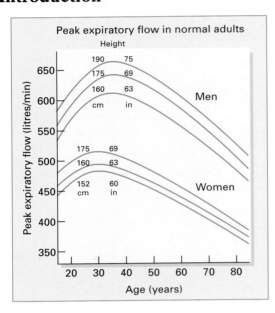

Peak expiratory flow in normal adults

The initial assessment of a patient with increased symptoms of asthma is important. Always err on the side of caution, because most problems result from undertreatment and failure to appreciate severity.

Monitor the peak flow rate and other signs before and after the first nebuliser treatment, and then as appropriate. In hospital, peak flow should be monitored at least four times daily for the duration of the stay.

Flow charts for management of acute asthma at home and in hospital are shown on pages 19 and 24. The various aspects of treatment are considered individually in this chapter.

β–stimulants

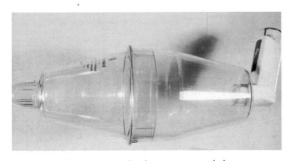

Volumatic spacer attached to a metered dose inhaler removes the importance of coordination between firing and inhalation.

Adrenaline has been used in the treatment of asthma for about 80 years. The specific β_2–stimulants such as salbutamol and terbutaline have replaced the earlier non-selective preparations both for regular and for acute use. There are no great differences in practice between the commonly used agents.

In acute asthma metered dose inhalers often lose their effectiveness. This is largely because of difficulties in the delivery of the drugs to the airways, and an alternative method of giving them is necessary—usually by nebuliser or intravenously. A temporary alternative if a nebuliser is not available is a large volume spacer (Nebuhaler or Volumatic). Like the nebuliser it has the advantage of removing the need to coordinate inhaler actuation and breathing. There is little or no difference in the effectiveness of drugs that are nebulised or given intravenously in acute severe asthma, so nebulisation is generally preferable.

It is helpful for general practitioners to have nebulisers available for acute asthmatic attacks. β–stimulants are best given by nebulisers driven by oxygen in acute asthma, as they may even worsen hypoxia slightly through an effect on the pulmonary vasculature. In general practice the use of oxygen as the driving gas is not usually practical. Domiciliary oxygen sets do not produce a flow rate adequate to drive most nebulisers, but if available they can be used with nasal spectacles during the nebulisation for a patient having an acute attack and by mask at other times. Many ambulance services are able to give nebulised drugs and oxygen during transfer to hospital.

In hospital, nebulisers used to treat asthmatic patients should be driven by oxygen except if the patient has chronic bronchitis and emphysema with carbon dioxide retention. The driving gas, flow rate,

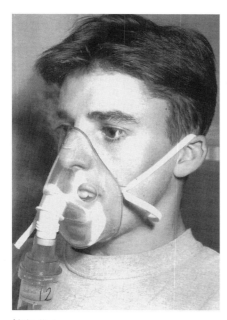

Nebuliser.

drug, diluent, and volume of fill should be clearly written on the prescription chart. Dilutions should always be done with saline to avoid bronchoconstriction from nebulisation of hypotonic solutions. There is no real advantage of nebulisation with a machine capable of producing intermittent positive pressure.

For adults the initial dose should be 5 mg salbutamol or its equivalent. This should be halved if the patient has ischaemic heart disease. It is essential to continue the intensive treatment after the first response; many of the problems in acute asthma arise because of complacency after the initial response to the first treatment. In severe attacks the nebulisation may need to be repeated every 15–30 minutes and can even be continuous.

If nebulised drugs are not effective then parenteral treatment should be considered. A reasonable plan is to give a β_2–agonist the first time, add an anticholinergic drug for the second nebulisation, and move to intravenous bronchodilators if there is no improvement. If life threatening features such as a raised carbon dioxide tension, an arterial oxygen tension < 8 kPa on oxygen, or a low pH are present, the intravenous agent should be used from the start.

The bronchodilator given parenterally in an acute attack can be β_2–agonist or aminophylline: there is little to choose between them. If the patient has been on theophylline and a level is not immediately available it is safer to use the β_2–stimulant. Salbutamol or terbutaline can be given intravenously over 10 minutes, or as an infusion, usually at 5–15 μg/minute. The adverse effects of tachycardia and tremor are much commoner after intravenous injection than after nebulisation.

Methylxanthines

Aminophylline is an effective bronchodilator in acute asthma but most studies have shown that it is no more effective than a β–stimulant given by nebulisation or intravenously. There are more problems with its use than with nebulised drugs and it should be reserved for patients with life-threatening features or who have failed to respond to nebulised drugs. Toxic effects are common and can occur with drug concentrations in or just above the therapeutic range. Concentrations are difficult to predict from the dose given because of individual differences in metabolic rate and interactions with drugs such as nicotine, cimetidine, erythromycin, and ciprofloxacin.

The position is further complicated if patients are already taking oral theophyllines. The usual starting dose for intravenous aminophylline is 250 mg given over 20–30 minutes. If the patient has taken oral theophylline or aminophylline in the previous 24 hours and a blood concentration is not available then the initial dose should be omitted or halved. A continuous infusion is then given at a rate of 0.5 mg/kg/hour, though this dose should be reduced if the patient also has kidney or liver disease. If intravenous treatment is necessary for more than 24 hours then blood concentrations should be measured and the rate adjusted as necessary.

> Theophylline clearance is reduced by:
> Erythromycin
> Cimetidine
> Allopurinol
> Frusemide
> Oral contraceptives
> Influenza vaccine

Corticosteroids

Corticosteroids are effective in preventing the development of acute asthma. Oral prednisolone should be given if control of asthma is deteriorating despite adequate bronchodilator treatment. A single oral dose of 20–40 mg prednisolone should be given each day for 7–14 days according to the speed of the response. The dose may then be stopped abruptly. If this opportunity is missed and an acute attack of asthma does develop corticosteroids are still an important element in treatment. Fatal attacks of asthma are associated with failure to prescribe any or adequate doses of corticosteroids. No noticeable response occurs for 4–6 hours, so corticosteroids should be started as early as possible and intensive bronchodilator treatment used while waiting for them to take effect.

In most cases oral corticosteroids are adequate, but when there are life threatening features intravenous hydrocortisone should be used in an initial dose of 200 mg followed by 200 mg six hourly for 24 hours. Prednisolone should be started at a dose of 30–60 mg daily whether or

> Airway responses to oral and intravenous corticosteroids come on slowly over several hours.

Treatment of acute asthma

not hydrocortisone is used (50 mg prednisolone is equivalent to 200 mg hydrocortisone). If the patient is first seen at home and transferred to hospital the first dose of corticosteroid should be given together with initial bronchodilator treatment before leaving home. When intensive initial treatment has been required prednisolone should be maintained at a dose of 30 mg/day for at least a week. Two to three weeks of treatment may be needed to obtain the maximal response with deflation to normal lung volumes and loss of excessive diurnal variations of peak flow. There are few side effects of such short courses of corticosteroids. Increased appetite, fluid retention, gastrointestinal upset, and psychological disturbance are most common. Exposure to herpes zoster may produce severe infections in susceptible individuals.

Anticholinergic agents

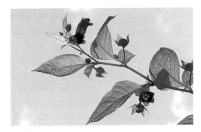

Atropa belladonna (deadly nightshade) which contains several anticholinergic substances.

At present ipratropium bromide is the only anticholinergic agent available in nebulised form in the United Kingdom. Nebulised ipratropium seems to be as effective as a nebulised β_2–stimulant in acute asthma. The dose of ipratropium is 500 μg and there are no problems with increased viscosity of secretions or mucociliary clearance at such doses. Ipratropium starts working more slowly than salbutamol: the peak response may not occur for 30–60 minutes. Adverse reactions such as paradoxical bronchoconstriction have been reported occasionally. These were related mainly to the osmolality of the solution or to the preservatives, and in the current preparations they have been corrected. Although the combination of β-stimulant and anticholinergic agents probably helps the initial improvement in acute attacks, β-stimulants are sufficient for most patients. Ipratropium can be added if the response to the first nebulisation is not considered adequate or if the initial assessment indicates that it is a very severe attack.

Oxygen

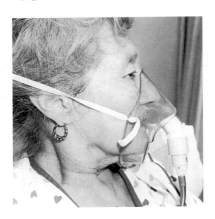

Acute severe asthma is always associated with hypoxia, although cyanosis develops late and is a grave sign. Death in asthma is caused by severe hypoxia, and oxygen should be given as soon as possible. It is very unusual to provoke carbon dioxide retention with oxygen treatment in asthma, and oxygen should therefore be given freely during transfer to hospital where blood gas measurement can be made. Masks can provide 40–50% oxygen. Nebulisers should be driven by oxygen whenever possible. In older subjects with exacerbation of chronic bronchitis and emphysema there is a potential danger of carbon dioxide retention. In these cases treatment should begin with 24% oxygen by Venturi mask until the results of blood gas measurements are available.

Fluid and electrolytes

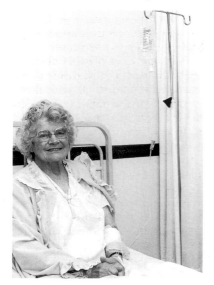

Patients with acute asthma tend to be dehydrated because they are often too breathless to drink and because fluid loss from the respiratory tract is increased. Dehydration increases the viscosity of mucus, making plugging of the airways more likely, so intravenous fluid replacement is often necessary. Three litres should be given during the first 24 hours if little oral fluid is being taken.

Increased alveolar ventilation, sympathomimetic drugs, and corticosteroids all tend to lower the serum potassium concentration. This is the most common disturbance of electrolytes in acute asthma, and the serum potassium concentration should be monitored and supplements given as necessary.

Antibiotics

Antibiotics should be reserved for patients with evidence of infection.

Upper respiratory tract infections are the commonest trigger factors for acute asthma and most of these are viral.

In only a few cases are exacerbations of asthma precipitated by bacterial infection. There is no evidence of benefit from the routine use of antibiotics, and these should be reserved for patients in whom there is presumptive evidence of infection such as fever, neutrophilia in the blood and sputum, and radiological changes. Although these features may occur in acute attacks without infection an antibiotic such as amoxycillin or erythromycin would be appropriate.

Controlled ventilation

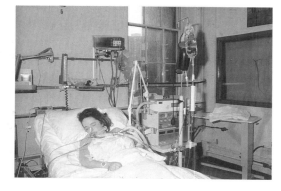

Patients with acute severe asthma who need hospital admission should be treated in an area able to deal with acute medical emergencies, with adequate nursing and medical supervision. If hypoxia is worsening, hypercapnia is present, or patients are exhausted or drowsy, then they should be nursed in an intensive care unit. Occasionally mechanical ventilation may be necessary for a short time while the treatment takes effect. It is usually needed because the patient becomes exhausted, and experience and careful observation are necessary to judge the right time to begin ventilatory support. Occasionally it can be avoided by the use of inspiratory positive airway pressure through a close fitting face mask, but patients may find it difficult to tolerate this treatment.

High inflation pressures and long expiratory times may make ventilation difficult in asthmatic patients, but most experienced units have good results provided that the decision to ventilate the patient is made electively and is not precipitated by respiratory arrest. When patients being mechanically ventilated fail to improve on adequate treatment bronchial lavage may occasionally be considered to reopen airways that have become plugged by mucus.

Other factors

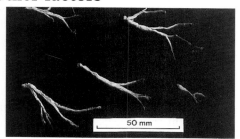

50 mm

Mucus plugs.

Most patients with acute severe asthma improve with these measures. Occasionally physiotherapy may be useful to help patients cough up thick plugs of sputum, but mucolytic agents to change the nature of the secretions do not help.

An episode of asthma is frightening, and the dangerous use of sedatives such as morphine was common before effective treatment became available. Unfortunately this practice still continues with occasional fatal consequences. Treatment of agitation should be aimed at reversing the asthma precipitating it, not at producing respiratory depression.

Discharge from hospital

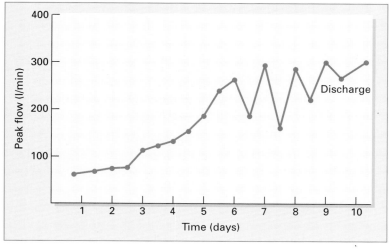

Peak flow during recovery from acute attack.

Discharge too early is associated with increased readmission and with mortality. Patients should have stopped nebuliser treatment and be using their own inhalers, with the proper technique checked, for at least 24 hours before discharge. Ideally peak flow should be above 75% of the patient's predicted or best reading and diurnal variability should be below 25%. A few patients may never lose their morning dips and may have to be discharged with them still present. For every patient the reason for the acute episode should be sought and appropriate changes made in their routine treatment and in their response to any deterioration to avoid similar attacks in the future. Patients with an acute attack of asthma should be looked after or at least seen by a physician with an interest in respiratory disease during their inpatient stay.

Subsequent management

> Good communication between hospital and general practitioner is essential.

Patients should not be discharged from hospital until their asthma is stable on the treatment that they will take at home, and they should leave with a plan of further management. This should include peak flow monitoring and a plan to respond to deteriorations in the control of their asthma. The general practitioner should be informed of the admission and the subsequent plans, and should see the patient within a week. The patient should return to the chest clinic within a month. Good communication between hospital and general practitioner is vital around this vulnerable period, and the telephone or fax machine may help.

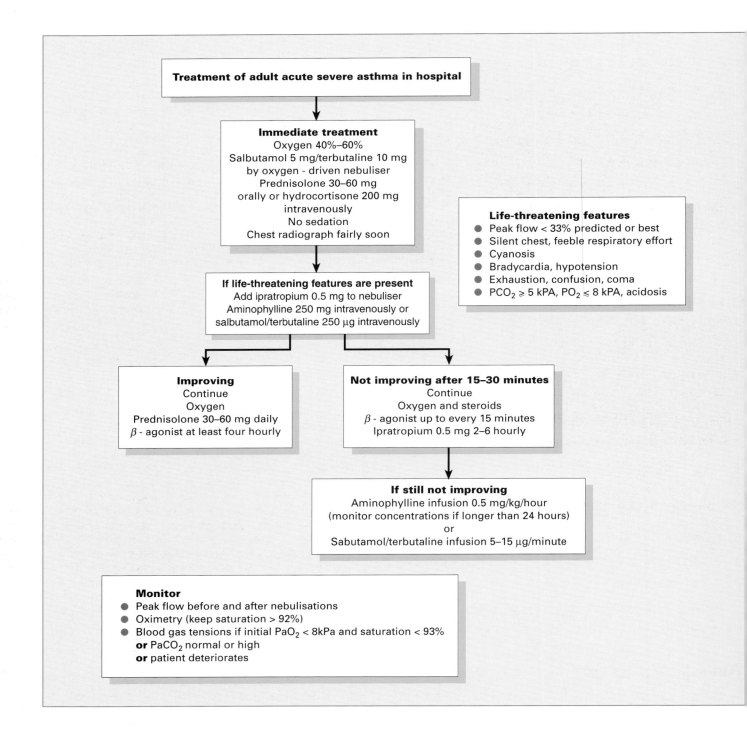

Treatment of adult acute severe asthma in hospital

Immediate treatment
Oxygen 40%–60%
Salbutamol 5 mg/terbutaline 10 mg
by oxygen - driven nebuliser
Prednisolone 30–60 mg
orally or hydrocortisone 200 mg
intravenously
No sedation
Chest radiograph fairly soon

If life-threatening features are present
Add ipratropium 0.5 mg to nebuliser
Aminophylline 250 mg intravenously or
salbutamol/terbutaline 250 µg intravenously

Life-threatening features
- Peak flow < 33% predicted or best
- Silent chest, feeble respiratory effort
- Cyanosis
- Bradycardia, hypotension
- Exhaustion, confusion, coma
- $PCO_2 \geq 5$ kPA, $PO_2 \leq 8$ kPA, acidosis

Improving
Continue
Oxygen
Prednisolone 30–60 mg daily
β - agonist at least four hourly

Not improving after 15–30 minutes
Continue
Oxygen and steroids
β - agonist up to every 15 minutes
Ipratropium 0.5 mg 2–6 hourly

If still not improving
Aminophylline infusion 0.5 mg/kg/hour
(monitor concentrations if longer than 24 hours)
or
Sabutamol/terbutaline infusion 5–15 µg/minute

Monitor
- Peak flow before and after nebulisations
- Oximetry (keep saturation > 92%)
- Blood gas tensions if initial PaO_2 < 8kPa and saturation < 93%
  or $PaCO_2$ normal or high
  or patient deteriorates

CHRONIC ASTHMA—GENERAL MANAGEMENT

General features

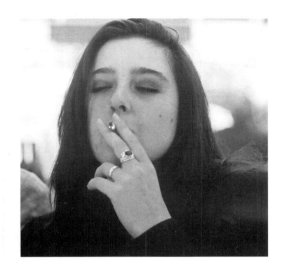

Obvious precipitating factors should be sought and avoided when practicable. This is possible for specific allergens such as animals and foods, but is not usually feasible with more widespread allergens such as pollens and house dust mites. A common non-specific stimulus is cigarette smoking. Up to a fifth of asthmatics continue to smoke and strenuous efforts should be made to discourage smoking in both asthmatic patients and their families. Precipitating factors should be carefully explored on one of the first visits but they should also be reassessed periodically.

Fortunately most asthmatic patients can have their disease controlled by safe drug treatment with minimal side effects. Education of the patient in understanding the disease and treatment is often helped by home peak flow recording and written explanations of the purpose and practical details of treatment. In particular, the differences between symptomatic bronchodilator treatment and regular maintenance treatment must be emphasised. It is all too common to find asthmatic patients using their dose of inhaled steroid or sodium cromoglycate only to treat an acute attack. Trained nurses can be helpful in continuing education and supervision.

Asthma clinics

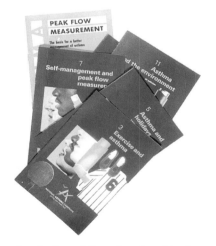

A selection of the educational leaflets produced by the National Asthma Campaign.

Many hospitals have concentrated their patients into specific asthma clinics for some years. The widespread interest in asthma clinics in general practice has been more recent. Training courses are available for nurses who take on such clinics. The clinics can be used to audit the treatment of asthmatic patients in a practice and ensure that all patients are encouraged to participate in their optimal management. Asthma clinics in general practice are best if they work with management guidelines and care plans. In some practices they are run by doctors, but in most cases it is nurses, who have more time to spend with each individual patient to go through inhaler techniques, understanding, and management plans. An interested doctor should be available for consultation and a close liaison should be built up with chest physicians at the local hospital.

Aims of management

> The ultimate goal is freedom from symptoms.

Persistent inflammation of the airways and increased bronchial reactivity have been recognised even in mild intermittent asthma. The inflammation can be targeted by drugs such as inhaled corticosteroids which reduce bronchial hyper–responsiveness, symptoms, and inflammatory infiltration of the airway. There has been a general move to be more aggressive in the treatment of asthma, the goal being freedom from symptoms rather than tolerance of shortness of breath

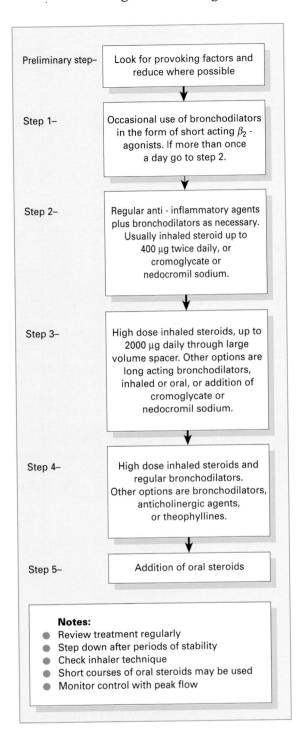

Preliminary step– | Look for provoking factors and reduce where possible

Step 1– | Occasional use of bronchodilators in the form of short acting β_2-agonists. If more than once a day go to step 2.

Step 2– | Regular anti - inflammatory agents plus bronchodilators as necessary. Usually inhaled steroid up to 400 µg twice daily, or cromoglycate or nedocromil sodium.

Step 3– | High dose inhaled steroids, up to 2000 µg daily through large volume spacer. Other options are long acting bronchodilators, inhaled or oral, or addition of cromoglycate or nedocromil sodium.

Step 4– | High dose inhaled steroids and regular bronchodilators. Other options are bronchodilators, anticholinergic agents, or theophyllines.

Step 5– | Addition of oral steroids

Notes:
- Review treatment regularly
- Step down after periods of stability
- Check inhaler technique
- Short courses of oral steroids may be used
- Monitor control with peak flow

and frequent need of bronchodilators. Regular treatment with inhaled β_2–agonists may even increase airway responsiveness but this is a controversial area. Most investigators have found a small increase in reactivity when regular β_2–agonists are taken for 4–6 weeks. A small number of longer term studies have suggested that the increase in reactivity does not progress any further. There has been a suggestion that regular use of β_2–agonists may be associated with a faster decline in lung function in asthmatic patients and the same association has been proposed for anticholinergic drugs. Anticholinergic agents have not been found to increase reactivity although when regular anticholinergic agents are stopped airway sensitivity to methacholine increases for about 24 hours. Theophyllines probably leave airway reactivity unchanged and have not been associated with accelerated decline in lung function, and there is renewed interest in their possible anti-inflammatory role. Some of these findings require confirmation, but they suggest that routine regular use of bronchodilators should be avoided. They should be used to treat symptoms and their use should be limited by the use of prophylactic agents. This approach fits with the various sets of guidelines published over the last few years.

Regular inhaled corticosteroids, however, decrease reactivity, as (probably) do sodium cromoglycate and nedocromil sodium. There is now evidence from studies of mild asthma that regular use of prophylactic agents reduces inflammation of the airways. The hope is that the reduction in the inflammation will prevent damage to the airway which would otherwise go on to produce irreversible obstruction. There is not yet any long term evidence for this, nor is there convincing evidence that inhaled steroids change the natural history of asthma in any other way. Reactivity is improved but not returned to normal.

Mild episodes of wheezing occurring once or twice a month can be controlled with inhaled β–stimulants. When attacks are more frequent regular treatment with inhaled steroids or sodium cromoglycate is necessary. Lack of adequate control should be sought by questions about sensitivity to irritants such as dust and smoke, about night–time symptoms, and by peak flow recording. Definite diurnal variation on peak flow readings or nocturnal waking indicates a high degree of reactivity of the airways and the need for vigorous treatment.

When chronic symptoms persist in the face of appropriate inhaled treatment a short course of oral corticosteroids often produces improvement which may last for many months after the course.

The aims of treatment are to avoid persistent symptoms and prevent acute attacks. In a variable disease such as asthma in which monitoring of the state of the disease is comparatively easy, the education and cooperation of the patient are vital parts of management. The patient should know how and when to take each treatment, broadly what each does, and exactly what to do in an exacerbation.

National and international consensus guidelines have been produced for the treatment of asthma. In the United Kingdom a number of groups combined to produce the first set of guidelines in 1990. A second version (including asthma in children) was published as a supplement to *Thorax* in 1993 (**48** suppl:S1–24). They produced a stepwise approach to the management of asthma which is summarised briefly above.

TREATMENT OF CHRONIC ASTHMA

β–stimulants

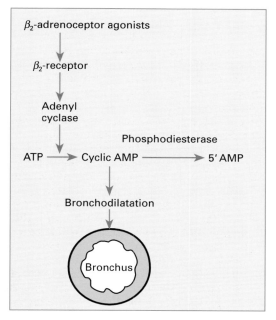

The first line of treatment of mild intermittent asthma is one of the selective β_2–stimulants taken by inhalation. β–stimulants are the most effective bronchodilator in asthma. They start to work quickly—salbutamol and terbutaline take effect within 15 minutes and last for four to six hours. If more than one daily dose is usually required then additional treatment must be considered. The dose response varies among patients as does the dose that will produce side effects, such as tremor. Patients should be taught to monitor their inhaler use and to understand that if they need it more or its effects lessen, these are danger signals. They indicate deterioration in asthmatic control and the need for further treatment.

Some patients worry that β–stimulants may become slightly less effective with time, particularly if the dose is high. There is little evidence of appreciable tachyphylaxis for the airway effects in asthmatics. If it exists it is a minor effect that is quickly reversed either by stopping the treatment temporarily or by taking corticosteroids. Tremor, palpitations, and muscle cramps may occur but are rarely troublesome if the drug is inhaled and these adverse effects outside the lung often become less of a problem with continued treatment.

The regular use of β–stimulants has in some studies been associated with increased bronchial reactivity, worsening asthma control, and accelerated decline of lung function. When the steps in the guidelines are followed, however, β–stimulants are not used regularly unless needed for control of symptoms.

Long acting β–stimulants

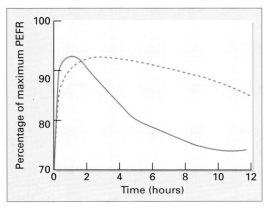

Bronchodilator response to oral salbutamol 200 μg (solid line) and inhaled salmeterol 50 μg (broken line).

Long acting preparations of oral β–agonists have been available for some years. They are effective in nocturnal asthma but are associated with more adverse effects than inhaled agents. The oral agent bambuterol, a prodrug of terbutaline, provides a newer longer acting alternative.

Long acting inhaled preparations are now available. They have an action that lasts at least 12 hours and can be used twice daily, or just at night if they are to prevent nocturnal problems. The protective effect against challenge may decline with prolonged use but the degree and duration of bronchodilator effect is maintained.

The precise place of the long acting agents is uncertain. There is a worry that their effectiveness and prolonged protection might mean that anti-inflammatory agents are neglected. This might allow underlying inflammation to continue so that a sufficient challenge might still lead to severe narrowing of the airway.

At present in asthma the long acting β–stimulants should be used only as an addition to inhaled corticosteroids. There is a debate about the dose of steroids achieved before the addition of long acting inhaled β–agonists. Some guidelines suggest a dose of 1000–2000 μg daily; others that are worried about the adverse effects of higher doses of inhaled corticosteroids suggest that drugs such as salmeterol should be added if control is inadequate with doses of corticosteroid below 1000 μg. Clinical studies have shown the effectiveness and safety of this approach.

Anticholinergic bronchodilators

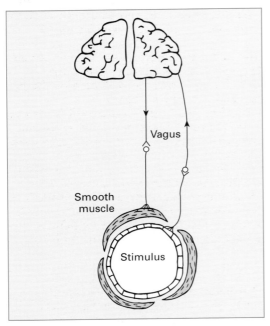

Anticholinergic agents block vagal efferent stimulation of bronchial smooth muscle.

Ipratropium bromide blocks the cholinergic bronchoconstrictor effect of the vagus nerve. Oxitropium bromide has a longer action, which makes it suitable for use two or three times a day. Anticholinergics are most effective in very young children and in older patients, and are generally more effective than β–stimulants in chronic bronchitis and emphysema. In most cases of asthma anticholinergic agents are less effective than β–stimulants, but they may supplement their effect if reversibility is incomplete. Anticholinergics take second place as bronchodilators in asthma unless tremor or tachycardia are troublesome side effects. If the response to a β–stimulant is inadequate then the technique of using the inhaler should be checked first. If this is satisfactory, evidence of an extra anticholinergic effect should be sought by measuring peak flow before and after inhalation of the β–agonist and then 30–60 minutes after adding the anticholinergic. At these doses there is no drying of secretions or interference with mucociliary clearance.

Methylxanthines

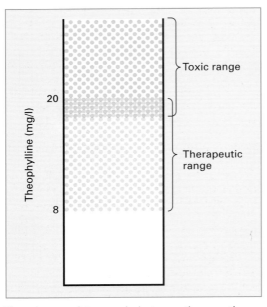

There is no safety margin between therapeutic and toxic ranges with theophylline.

Theophylline is an effective bronchodilator and may also have anti-inflammatory actions. Its safety margin is low compared with other bronchodilators which can be given by inhalation. Individual differences in the doses required are high, so that it is necessary to monitor treatment by blood concentrations. Inhaled treatment with β–agonists is preferable, but slow release theophyllines are an alternative to long acting β–agonists for nocturnal symptoms. Absorption of aminophylline from suppositories is much less predictable and they are best avoided.

The commonest side effects of theophylline are nausea, vomiting, and abdominal discomfort, but headache, malaise, fast pulse rate, and fits also occur, sometimes without early warning from gastrointestinal symptoms. The dose of theophylline should start at around 7 mg/kg/day in divided doses, and build up. All patients taking theophylline should have their peak concentrations monitored and doses adjusted until they are between 8 and 18 mg/l (40–90 μmol/l). Above 20 mg/l toxic effects are unacceptably high, although 15%–30% of patients will have gastrointestinal effects with smaller doses. Theophylline clearance is increased by smoking, alcohol consumption, and enzyme inducing drugs such as phenytoin, rifampicin, and barbiturates. Clearance will be decreased and blood concentrations rise if it is given at the same time as cimetidine, ciprofloxacin, or erythromycin, and in the presence of heart failure, liver impairment, or pneumonia.

There is in vitro evidence that theophyllines have an anti-inflammatory effect even at low doses. Further work is needed on the clinical use of low dose theophylline as an anti-inflammatory agent.

Sodium cromoglycate and nedocromil sodium

Must be used regularly for at least 4–8 weeks before being dismissed as ineffective.

Sodium cromoglycate blocks bronchoconstrictor responses to challenge by exercise and antigens. The original proposed mechanism of stabilisation of mast cells may not be the main mechanism of its action in asthma. It can be used as the first line prophylactic agent if control of asthma requires more than an occasional inhalation of β–agonist, and success is most likely with young atopic asthmatic patients but may occur at any age. Sodium cromoglycate used to be given as a dry powder in Spincaps but metered dose inhalers delivering 5 mg/

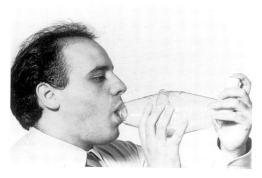

The large volume spacers overcome problems with coordination of inhaler firing and inspiration. They reduce oropharyngeal deposition of aerosol and improve delivery to the lung.

actuation are more convenient and just as effective. Occasionally patients develop reflex bronchoconstriction in response to the irritant effects of the dry powder, and if they do, they should try changing to a metered dose inhaler or using a dose of inhaled β–agonist 10–15 minutes earlier.

Other adverse reactions to sodium cromoglycate are rare. Other mast cell stabilisers have been disappointing, possibly because of the additional effects of cromoglycate. The oral agent ketotifen produces drowsiness in 10% of patients and has little activity.

Cromoglycate should not be dismissed as ineffective until it has been tried for at least 4–8 weeks and it must be used regularly. It has no place in the treatment of acute exacerbations of asthma and may even increase narrowing of the airways by its irritant effect.

Nedocromil sodium has the same properties as sodium cromoglycate but may have an additional anti-inflammatory effect on the airway epithelium. It is probably more useful than sodium cromoglycate in older patients although it is less effective than inhaled corticosteroids in most subjects. It may be tried as a first line in patients with mild disease or as an addition to inhaled corticosteroids when control of symptoms is inadequate.

Inhaled corticosteroids

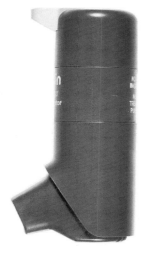

The autohaler device is triggered by inspiratory airflow and is available for β–agonists, anticholinergics and corticosteroids.

Steroids may be given by metered dose inhaler or dry powder devices, and the dose should be adjusted to give optimum control. The two commonest inhaled steroids, beclomethasone dipropionate and budesonide, are roughly equivalent in dose. The newer agent fluticasone seems to have less systemic effects at the same dose and it can be used at half the dose of beclomethasone dipropionate with the same therapeutic effect.

Inhaled steroids may be given twice daily with no problems apart from occasional oropharyngeal candidiasis or a husky voice until a daily dose above the equivalent of 1000 μg beclomethasone dipropionate is reached. At higher doses there may be biochemical evidence of suppression of the hypothalamic-pituitary-adrenal axis, even with inhaled steroids, but this is not a particular problem in adults.

With doses of more than 1000 μg daily of budesonide or beclomethasone there are metabolic effects including an increase in the concentration of osteocalcin, a marker of increased bone turnover. There is some evidence of skin thinning and purpura even in patients who have not had appreciable doses of oral steroids. Doses over 2000 μg daily are not often used but when necessary nebulised budesonide may be a convenient strategy. A large volume spacer should be used at doses above 800 μg daily to reduce the pharyngeal deposition of metered dose inhalers.

Doses of inhaled steroids should be taken regularly to be effective. There is evidence that doubling the regular dose when an upper respiratory infection develops reduces the risk of problems from an exacerbation of asthma.

The main difficulties in the use of inhaled corticosteroids are the patients' worries about the use of steroids and the difficulties of ensuring that patients take regular medication even when they are well. These problems are increased by the move to use inhaled corticosteroids earlier in asthma and to try to achieve a level of control that is free of symptoms.

There is a suggestion that control is achieved more easily by the use of a high dose of inhaled steroids at the start then a reduction as control is achieved. When asthma is under control the next decision is how long to maintain the inhaled steroids. The dose should be reviewed regularly and if doses above 1000 μg daily have been necessary these should be reduced when possible. Most physicians like to have complete asthma control for 6–12 months before trying to stop prophylaxis completely.

Side effects of inhaled corticosteroids

Established:
- Oropharyngeal candida
- Dysphonia
- Irritation and cough

Suggested at high dose:
- Adrenal suppression
- Reduced growth in children
- Purpura and thinning of skin
- Osteoporosis
- Cataract

Oral corticosteroids

Long term corticosteroids should be used only if other drugs have failed.

Occasional asthmatic patients have to take long term oral corticosteroids but this should be only after the failure of vigorous treatment with other drugs, and the symptoms or risks of the disease must be balanced against the adverse effects of long term treatment with oral corticosteroids. It is important to remember that, in contrast,

Treatment of chronic asthma

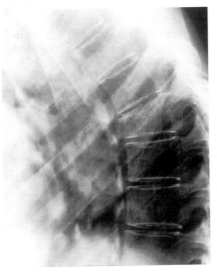

Osteoporotic collapse of a thoracic vertebra in a patient taking oral steroids.

short courses of oral steroids for exacerbations of symptoms and inhaled steroids have few serious problems.

Short courses of oral steroids may be stopped abruptly or tailed off over a few days. Low concentrations of cortisol and adrenocorticotropic hormone (ACTH) are found for just 2–3 days after 40 mg prednisolone daily for three weeks, but clinical problems with responses to stress or exacerbations of asthma do not occur. An appropriate course would be 25–40 mg prednisolone daily for 14 days. Most asthmatic patients can be taught to keep such a supply of steroids at home and to use them according to their individual management plan when predetermined signs of deteriorating control occur.

If patients require long term oral steroids, they should be settled on a regimen of treatment on alternate days whenever possible. The goal is always to establish control with other treatment which will allow the discontinuation of the oral steroids. Inhaled steroids in moderate to high doses should be maintained to keep the oral dose as low as possible. Alternative preparations such as ACTH and triamcinolone are less flexible and give no appreciable benefit in terms of adrenal suppression.

A small proportion of asthmatic patients are fully or partially resistant to corticosteroids. They form a particularly difficult group to treat.

Desensitisation and avoidance of allergens

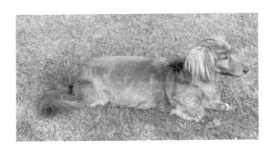

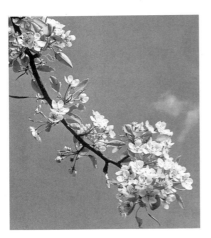

As discussed in chapter 4, the results of trials of desensitisation and avoidance of allergens have been disappointing. Some patients have obvious precipitating factors—in particular, animals—and avoidance is helpful, but there are usually other unknown precipitating factors. More common are patients with reactive airways who are also sensitive to pollens, house dust mite, and other allergens. Such stimuli are almost impossible to avoid completely in everyday life, although symptoms improve with rigorous measures such as admission to a dust free environment in hospital. Nevertheless it is sensible to try to reduce the exposure to known allergens as much as possible. In children at risk of asthma it may be particularly important to limit their exposure to potential allergic problems.

There is some evidence that desensitisation is beneficial in patients with asthma who are sensitive to pollens, and that repeated courses increase the improvement. Controlled studies in adults sensitive to house dust mites have shown no benefit from desensitisation. Several studies in children have suggested some benefit, but these were highly selected patients, and it is unusual to find asthmatic patients with a single sensitivity. The degree of control produced by desensitisation can usually be achieved with simple, safe, inhaled drugs.

There is little sound evidence to support desensitisation to other agents in asthmatic patients. In particular, cocktails produced from the results of skin tests or radioallergosorbent tests are not a valid form of treatment. Local reactions to desensitising agents are common and more generalised reactions and even death can occur. Most deaths are related to errors in the injection schedule and inadequate supervision after injections. Desensitisation should be undertaken only where appropriate facilities for resuscitation are available.

One area where desensitisation is appropriate is in sensitivity to insect venom which results in anaphylaxis rather than asthma. Aspirin induced asthma may respond to careful oral desensitisation.

Other drug treatments

Preparations which combine a prophylactic agent and a short acting bronchodilator do not fit into care guidelines. Inhaled bronchodilators should be used as necessary.

Some fixed dose combinations are available for the treatment of asthma, but they have little to commend them. Combinations of bronchodilators may be used when such treatment has been shown to be appropriate in drug and in dose. This is unusual in asthma.

Combinations of bronchodilator and prophylactic drug do not fit easily into most guidelines for the treatment of asthma. It has been suggested that they may improve compliance with the prophylaxis, but this is not certain. They take away flexibility of treatment. Several oral combinations are available, often with small doses of theophylline, ephedrine, and barbiturate. There is no indication for such preparations.

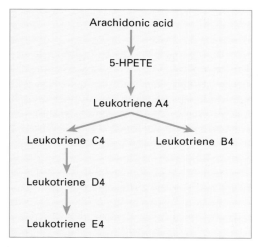

Arachidonic acid

↓

5-HPETE

↓

Leukotriene A4

Leukotriene C4   Leukotriene B4

↓

Leukotriene D4

↓

Leukotriene E4

Leukotriene antagonists are being developed and may act as alternative prophylactic agents in asthma.

Other drugs such as α–stimulants, antihistamines, and calcium antagonists may have some effect, but have not found a role in treatment. Newer antagonists to leukotrienes, platelet activating factor, and other mediators are under trial.

When large doses of corticosteroids are necessary, or in patients who fail to respond to steroids, other agents have been tried. Methotrexate, gold, and cyclosporin have shown evidence of benefit, mainly in reducing the dose of steroids necessary for control. All are associated with substantial potential side effects.

Other treatments

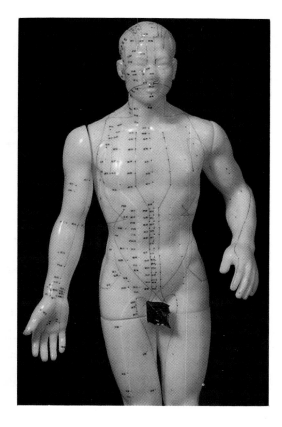

There have been dramatic claims for the benefit of yoga, hypnosis, and acupuncture but few have been confirmed in controlled trials. Relaxation may help to reduce the anxiety and hyperventilation which can exacerbate asthma. Such techniques may be useful in dealing with exacerbations. Patients' worries about the future course of asthma and its dangers should be explored and dealt with.

Ionisation of inspired air may have a small effect on lung function and may attenuate the response to exercise, but such effects are minimal and not achieved by home ionisers. Some herbal remedies may contain useful ingredients which need investigation. Some contain conventional agents which are not standardised, however, and some even contain corticosteroids and have produced the expected side effects.

METHODS OF DELIVERING DRUGS

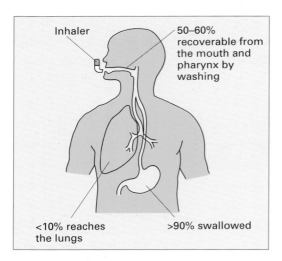

Various devices and formulations have been developed to deliver drugs efficiently, minimise side effects, and simplify use. With the range of devices now available it is possible for nearly all patients to have their drugs by inhalation. In some circumstances oral treatment is needed and it can be given by slow acting or sustained release preparations.

Metered dose inhalers

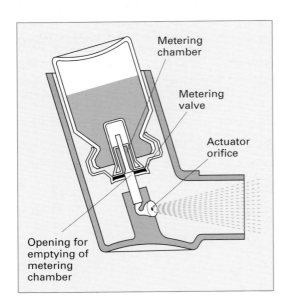

Inhalers deliver the drug directly to the airways. A metered dose inhaler used properly deposits about 10% of the drug into the airways below the larynx. Nearly all the rest of the drug gets no further than the oropharynx and is swallowed. This swallowed portion may be absorbed from the gastrointestinal tract but drugs such as inhaled corticosteroids are largely removed by first pass metabolism in the liver. Absorption directly from the lung bypasses liver metabolism.

An important point in the prescription of inhalation treatment is the instruction of the patient in the technique. A metered dose inhaler should be shaken, and then fired into the mouth shortly after the start of a slow full inspiration. At full inflation the breath should be held for 10 seconds. The technique should be checked periodically. About a quarter of patients have difficulty using a metered dose inhaler and the problems increase with age. Arthritic patients who find it hard to exert the pressure on the inhaler may be helped by a "Haleraid" device which responds to squeezing, or they can be given a dry powder system.

Current metered dose inhalers contain freons as propellants. Medicines make up a tiny percentage of total freon use but it is likely to be restricted over the next few years. Some countries have already stopped the use of inhalers containing harmful freons and pharmaceutical companies are working on alternative propellant vehicles which will be "environmentally friendly".

Breath actuated inhalers

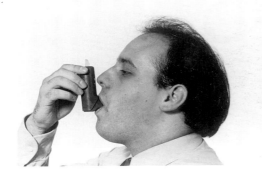

Breath actuated inhalers are available for most classes of drug. The valve on the inhaler is actuated as the patient breathes in. The devices respond to a low inspiratory flow rate and are useful for those who have difficulty coordinating actuation and breathing, and generally they seem to increase lung deposition of drug. They require a propellant similar to that used in a standard inhaler.

Extension tubes

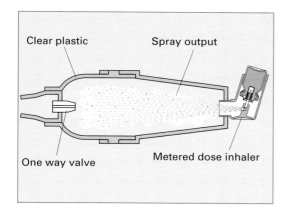

Clear plastic

Spray output

One way valve

Metered dose inhaler

The coordination of firing and inspiration becomes slightly less important when a short extension tube is used. This may help if problems are minor but a larger reservoir removes the need for coordination of breathing and actuation. The inhaler is fixed into the chamber and the breath is taken from a one way valve at the other end of the chamber. Inhalation should be within 30 seconds of the actuation of the inhaler. Pharyngeal deposition is greatly reduced as the faster particles strike the walls of the chamber, not the mouth, and evaporation of propellant from the larger slower particles produces a small sized aerosol which penetrates further out into the lungs and deposits a greater proportion of drug beyond the larynx. This reduces the risk of oral candidiasis and dysphonia with inhaled corticosteroids and reduces potential problems with systemic absorption from the gastrointestinal tract. They should be used routinely when doses of inhaled steroid of more than 800 μg daily are given by metered dose inhaler.

The device is cumbersome, but this is no great disadvantage for corticosteroid treatment which is usually given only twice a day. These chambers can be used for all types of inhalers and have proved useful as a substitute for a nebuliser in acute asthma.

Dry powder inhalers

Dry powder inhalers of various types are available for β–agonists, sodium cromoglycate, corticosteroids and in some countries, anticholinergic agents. Because inspiratory airflow releases the fine powder many problems of coordination are avoided, and there are none of the environmental worries of metered dose inhalers. The dry powder makes some patients cough, however. The problems of reloading for each dose have been eased by the development of multiple dose units with up to 200 doses. Dry powder devices such as the Turbohaler increase lung deposition above 20% of the dose and may allow a reduction in the prescribed dose.

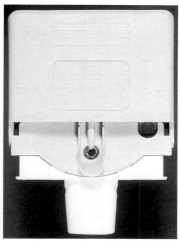

Dry powder diskhalers are available for inhaled steroids and β–agonists.

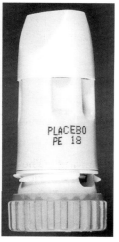

PLACEBO
PE 18

The Turbohaler contains multiple doses of dry powder for inhalation and is available for corticosteroids and β–agonists.

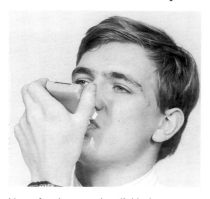

Use of a dry powder diskhaler.

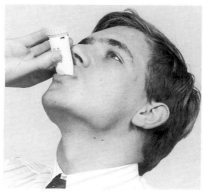

Use of a dry powder Turbohaler.

Methods of delivering drugs

Nebulisers

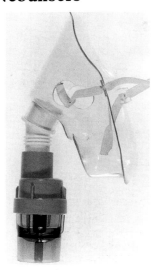

Nebulisers can be driven by compressed gas (jet nebuliser) or an ultrasonically vibrating crystal (ultrasonic nebuliser). They provide a way of giving inhaled drugs to those unable to use any other device—for example, the very young, or in acute attacks when inspiratory flow is limited. Nebulisers also offer a convenient way of delivering a higher dose to the airways. Generally, about 12% of the drug leaving the chamber enters the lungs but most of the dose stays in the apparatus or is wasted in expiration. Delivery depends on the type of nebuliser chamber, the flow rate at which it is driven, and the volume in the chamber. In most cases flow rates of less than 6 l/minute in a jet nebuliser give too large a particle and nebulise too slowly. Some chambers have a reservoir and valve system to reduce loss to the surrounding room during expiration.

Tablets and syrups

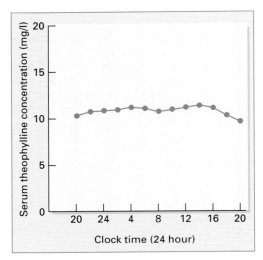

Steady theophylline concentrations in the therapeutic range can be obtained with twice daily slow release preparations.

Tablets and syrups are available for oral use. This route is necessary for theophyllines which cannot be inhaled effectively. Very young children who are unable to inhale drugs can take the sugar free liquid preparations. Slow release tablets are used when a prolonged action is needed, particularly for nocturnal asthma in which theophyllines have proved helpful. Various slow release mechanisms or long acting drugs have been developed to maintain even blood concentrations.

Injections and infusions

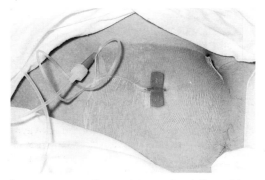

In severe cases β–agonists can be delivered by subcutaneous infusion.

Injections are used for the treatment of acute attacks. Subcutaneous injections may be useful in emergencies when nebulisers are unavailable. Occasional patients with severe chronic asthma seem to benefit from the high levels of β–stimulant obtained with subcutaneous infusion through a portable pump. Rates may need to be adjusted depending on severity. The infusion site is changed by the patient every 1–3 days.

ASTHMA IN CHILDREN: PREVALENCE AND PROSPECTS FOR PREVENTION

Asthma on the increase

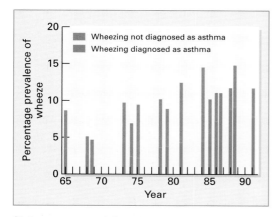

Sixteen surveys of the 12 month prevalence of (a) wheezing not diagnosed as asthma and (b) wheezing diagnosed as asthma in children, 1965–91.

Studies published in the early 1980s that emphasised the morbidity of asthma and its underdiagnosis have led to wider recognition of the condition in children. Even allowing for this change in "diagnostic labelling" there has been a remarkable increase in the prevalence of childhood asthma over the past 15–20 years. For example the National Study of Health and Growth suggested that the incidence of asthma that caused symptoms in children on most days went up by about 5% a year between 1973 and 1986. Over the same period hospital admission rates doubled in children of school age and quadrupled in preschool children. About 40 children die of asthma each year and mortality shows no sign of declining. When asthma deaths have been investigated the one consistent preventable factor has been undertreatment, either of the last attack or in the long term.

Childhood asthma is a serious public health problem. More than half of all cases of asthma at any age present before the age of 10 years. Currently over 30% of children experience a wheezing illness during the first few years of life and 10%–20% will have asthma diagnosed in later childhood. More absence from school is caused by asthma than any other chronic condition; 30% of asthmatic children miss more than three weeks of schooling each year. Asthma influences educational attainment even in children of above average intelligence, the extent of this adverse effect being related to the severity of the disease.

These disappointing figures apply over a period of time during which there have been many new developments for the treatment of asthmatic children. The specific β-adrenergic bronchodilators, sodium cromoglycate, controlled release bronchodilators, ketotifen, and inhaled steroids have become available together with new delivery systems for both inhaled and oral antiasthma drugs. A review of prescribing practices suggested, however, that while prescriptions for bronchodilator drugs have steadily increased there is still a reluctance among doctors to prescribe, and among the parents of young asthmatic children to give, regular preventive medication.

Airway inflammation

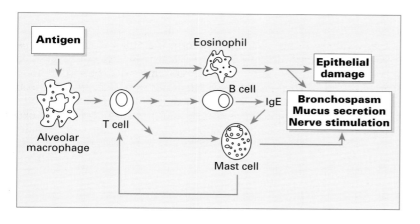

The airways of children who die of asthma show an intense inflammatory response. Fibreoptic bronchoscopy and the safe techniques for bronchial biopsy and bronchoalveolar lavage that have been developed have shown that there is an inflammatory cellular infiltrate in the airways of asthmatic adults even when they are free of symptoms. This has led to the concept that all asthma is a chronic inflammatory disorder. Eosinophils and mast cells are the important effector cells, the inflammatory process being modulated by T lymphocytes and macrophages and amplified by neural mechanisms.

Diagnosis and the choice of treatment
depends on clinical judgement based on
the nature, frequency, and severity of
symptoms combined with physiological
assessment of airway function.

Indirect evidence of an inflammatory process in the airways of young children has come from measurement of markers of inflammation in the blood, but few histological studies have been done in children. We do not know how or when the inflammatory process starts, at what stage it becomes irreversible, or even whether the same type of inflammatory response occurs in all young wheezy children. No component of the inflammatory process can be used as a diagnostic test for childhood asthma or as a reliable way to assess response to treatment.

Children at risk

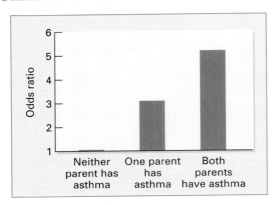

Odds ratios for asthma in offspring.

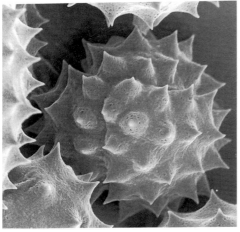

Pollen grains.

Why has there been a rise in the prevalence of childhood asthma and is there anything that can be done to reverse the trend? The development of asthma is subject to genetic influence, which is illustrated by its increased prevalence in children of atopic parents. The life prevalence in childhood increases from about 20% to more than half if one or both parents have asthma or hay fever. The risk seems to increase irrespective of the parents' "atopic disease," which suggests that the general susceptibility to atopy is important. Studies in twins, however, have suggested that genetic factors account for only 60%–70% of asthma. In other words, environmental influence is also important. This encourages the prospect for prevention if either adverse factors in the environment can be removed or the airway response to them modulated. But first it is necessary to identify infants who are particularly at risk.

If the selection of children for preventive measures is based on family history most children at risk would receive them but about half of the children would not have developed asthma anyway. IgE production is genetically dictated and a high concentration of IgE in cord blood to some extent predicts susceptibility to asthma. The sensitivity is quite good—most children with high cord blood IgE concentrations will develop atopic illnesses—but the specificity is poor in that it identifies only about 40% of children who subsequently develop asthma. Genetic predisposition is influenced by gender; asthma generally, and severe asthma in particular, is more common among boys. Children with atopic disease are more likely to have an allergic mother than an allergic father, so boys with asthmatic mothers and a raised cord blood IgE concentration would be a very high risk group. The trouble is that if all these criteria were taken as the indication for preventive measures, only a small proportion of the total number of children at risk of asthma would receive attention. There is as yet no satisfactory way of predicting the onset of asthma in childhood with both high sensitivity and specificity.

Prospects for prevention

Atmospheric pollution

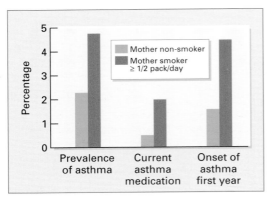

Maternal smoking and asthma in children aged 0–5 years (based on National Health Interview Survey, 1981, n = 4331).

Young children spend most of their time indoors so indoor pollution is likely to have a greater influence on the development of asthma than outdoor pollution. The most important cause of pollution indoors is tobacco smoke and there is abundant evidence that parental, and particularly maternal, smoking increases the prevalence of childhood asthma. Children whose mothers smoke more than 10 cigarettes a day are twice as likely to develop asthma as those whose mothers are non-smokers. Maternal smoking in pregnancy is associated with raised IgE concentrations in cord blood and increased airway reactivity in early infancy. Because cigarette smoking is harmful in many other ways it is undoubtedly justifiable to encourage parents to stop smoking. Indeed, it would be unethical not to do so.

Some epidemiological studies have suggested that outdoor air pollution increases the severity of childhood asthma. For example, children living in polluted areas of Spain and Scandinavia have more frequent attacks of asthma than those living in unpolluted regions. So far it has proved impossible to define the effects of the individual components of outdoor atmospheric pollution.

> The evidence that outdoor pollution has an impact on the prevalence of asthma is less compelling than that for cigarette smoke.

Exposure to allergens in early infancy

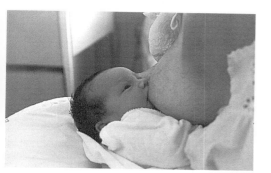

There may be a critical period in early life when exposure to allergens leads to sensitisation rather than tolerance, increasing the risk of asthma. Over the past 50 years many studies have investigated the influence of breast feeding and restriction of dietary allergens on the development of asthma. About equal numbers have shown a beneficial effect and no advantage. While the debate continues the other advantages of breast milk should persuade us to continue advising breast feeding in atopic families.

Inhaled allergens have a greater influence on the development of asthma than dietary allergens. Studies of month of birth have suggested that exposure to pollen or house dust mite allergens during the first three months of life increases the risk of sensitisation. A prospective study of children with atopic parents showed that the probability of asthma persisting to the age of 11 years was increased fivefold if the children were exposed to high levels of the major house dust mite antigen Der p 1 in early childhood. The mechanism by which sensitisation occurs is not yet understood; IgE production is controlled by regulatory T cells but we know relatively little about the cellular responses to inhaled allergens in early life. Whatever the mechanism, it must now be asked if asthma can be modified or prevented by avoidance of house dust mites during infancy. A study currently being conducted on the Isle of Wight has found that the prevalence of wheezing during the first year of life in children of atopic parents was reduced by avoiding a combination of dietary and inhaled allergens but it remains to be seen whether this difference persists as the children grow older.

ASTHMA IN CHILDREN: PATTERNS OF ILLNESS AND DIAGNOSIS

Wheezing in infancy

Factors that influence wheezing in infancy

Prenatal
- Airway size—Gender
- Maternal smoking
- Prematurity
- Parental atopy, allergen exposure

Postnatal
- Viral infection
- Allergen exposure
- Pollution—indoor/outdoor

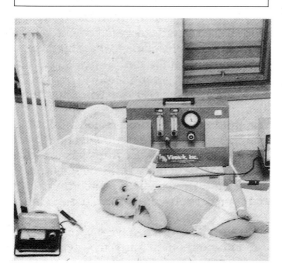

Infants are particularly prone to wheezing illnesses. Their airways are narrow and their compliant chest walls allow the airways to collapse towards the end of expiration. In the past it was thought that in early childhood the lung airways might be deficient in smooth muscle and β-adrenoreceptors. This is not the case, because infants show a bronchoconstrictor response to histamine that can be prevented with salbutamol. There are several different categories of wheezy infant. Many babies have repeated episodes of wheezing apparently associated with viral respiratory tract infections. The mechanism by which this happens is still not fully understood but genetic constitution and environmental influences in early life may predispose to wheezing by causing changes in airway calibre or in lung function. For example, wheezy lower respiratory illnesses are more common among boys, among infants of parents who smoke, and among babies born prematurely who have needed prolonged positive pressure ventilation. It has been postulated that pre-existing factors other than asthma which cause narrowing of the airways account for more than a half of the wheezing developed by infants. Environmental factors may operate prenatally as well as postnatally; changes in lung function have been observed in four week old infants whose mothers have smoked during pregnancy.

About 1% of infants are admitted to hospital with acute viral bronchiolitis. Recurrent cough and wheezing commonly follow, but in most cases stop before school age. About 40% of babies with atopic eczema also develop recurrent wheezing and there is a strong association between a family history of atopic disease and wheezing in early childhood. Only a small proportion of children who wheeze in infancy continue to wheeze throughout childhood, but on the other hand most children who develop severe asthma start having symptoms during their early life.

Changes with age

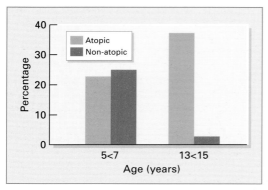

Atopy in children with bronchial hyper-reactivity.

During preschool years viral infections, exercise, and emotional upset are common triggers of asthma. Young children contract six to eight viral upper respiratory tract infections each year so it is not surprising that these infections are more common precipitants of asthma in children than in adults. Asthmatic children tend to have more symptoms during the winter than the summer, probably because viral respiratory infections are more common in winter and because exercise induced asthma is more likely to develop outdoors in cold weather.

A recent population study in New Zealand reported that as children grew older bronchial reactivity decreased. Judged by the response to inhaled histamine the number of children with hyper-responsive airways halved between the ages of 6 and 12. In contrast the number of atopic children doubled. Of those between the ages of 5 and 7 who had evidence of bronchial reactivity about half were atopic and about half were not; of the children aged 13 with bronchial hyper-responsiveness

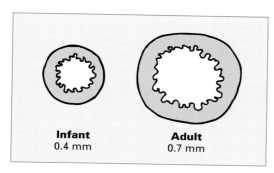

Diameter of bronchioles.

over 90% were atopic. These results support the clinical observations that non-specific factors, notably viral infections and exercise, are important triggers of asthma during pre-school years and allergic triggers assume greater importance as children grow older. The increase in airway size with growth and the apparent spontaneous decline in airway responsiveness with age parallels the improvement in asthma in non-atopic children. The signs of atopy on the other hand are linked with persistence of asthma into the second decade of life.

Mortality from childhood asthma is highest between the ages of 10 and 15 years. Paradoxically it is also the time when many asthmatic children become symptom free. The idea that "most children grow out of their asthma" has been refuted by recent studies which have suggested that less than half of asthmatic children become and remain symptom free in adulthood. About 30% of those who do lose their symptoms in adolescence have some recurrence in early adult life.

Diagnosis

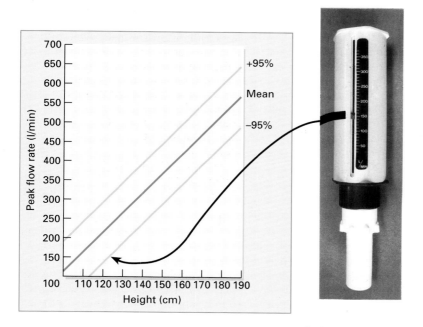

Most recurrent wheezing in childhood is caused by asthma, and the diagnosis can usually be made from a carefully taken history. In school age children there is little difficulty in recognising asthma. Preschool children sometimes present with cough alone. The characteristics that suggest asthma are that cough or wheezing is episodic, worse at night, after exercise, or exposure to allergens, accompanies viral respiratory tract infections, and occurs in children with a family history of atopic disease. Asthmatic babies sometimes have attacks of breathlessless without obvious wheezing. Occasionally in older children the only feature is breathlessness on exercise. Some asthmatic children produce large amounts of bronchial secretions—so-called hypersecretory asthma. Increased production of mucus is associated with a productive cough, airway plugging, and areas of collapse in the chest radiograph. These children may be misdiagnosed as having recurrent lower respiratory tract infection.

Certain features suggest that the cough or wheezing may be caused by factors other than asthma. These include onset in the newborn period, chronic diarrhoea or failure to thrive, recurrent infections, choking or difficulty with swallowing, mediastinal or focal abnormalities in the chest radiograph, and the presence of cardiovascular abnormalities.

When possible the diagnosis should be confirmed by lung function testing. This can be done at any age, but in infants and very young children the facilities are available only in specialised centres. From the age of 3–4 years children can use a peak flow meter, and the peak flow reading can be compared with a range of values related to the child's height. A normal peak flow reading at one examination does not of course exclude asthma, and several recordings made at home may be more valuable. Occasionally an exercise test or therapeutic trial is necessary to confirm the diagnosis. Measurement of total IgE concentration will ascertain only whether the child is atopic, and a chest radiograph is more useful to look for other causes of wheezing than to diagnose asthma.

Historically asthma has carried a certain stigma; an image of a small, thin child who is breathless and ill. Perhaps for this reason there has sometimes been a reluctance to tell parents that their child has asthma. As long as appropriate explanation and management follows, parents' anxiety is much more likely to be relieved than increased by being told the diagnosis.

Other causes of wheezing in children

Bronchiolitis
Inhalation:
    Foreign body
    Milk
Cystic fibrosis
Tuberculosis
Bronchomalacia
Tracheal or bronchial stenosis
Vascular rings
Mediastinal masses

Assessment of severity

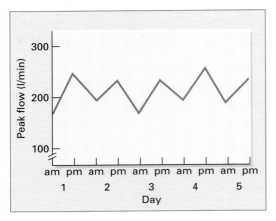

Ideally the management of asthma should include serial measurement of markers of disease activity, but as yet there are none which can be applied to the clinical care of asthmatic children. Evaluation of severity and response to treatment has therefore to be made by clinical assessment complemented when possible by measurements of lung function. A sound approach is to classify the asthma as mild, moderate, or severe; to base the initial treatment regimen on this assessment; and then decide at regular reviews whether there is scope to reduce, or need to increase, medication.

For asthma to be categorised as mild, symptomatic episodes should occur less frequently than once a month and usually be provoked by viral respiratory tract infections. Symptoms do not interfere with daytime activity or sleep. There is a good response to bronchodilator treatment, and lung function returns to normal between attacks.

Children with moderate asthma have some symptoms several days a week and have attacks of asthma more than once a month but less than once a week. There is no chest deformity and growth is unaffected. Attacks may be triggered by viral infection, allergens, exercise, cigarette smoke, climatic changes, and emotional upset.

The third category, severe asthma, is the least common. The children have troublesome symptoms on most days, wake frequently with asthma at night, miss at lot of schooling, and are unable to participate fully in school activities. Many have chest deformities and growth may be retarded.

Some children do not fit any of these categories. Seasonal asthma caused by allergy to grass pollen generally affects older children. A few children have sudden very severe attacks of asthma which result in admission to hospital and may be life threatening, separated by long periods without symptoms during which their lung function returns to normal. This last group are very difficult to treat.

	Mild	Moderate	Severe
Frequency of attacks	<1/month	>1/month	>1/week
Lung function between attacks	Normal	Often abnormal	Always abnormal
Chest deformity	No	No	Yes
Growth	Normal	Normal	Retarded
Response to bronchodilator	Good	Variable	Poor

ASTHMA IN CHILDREN: TREATMENT

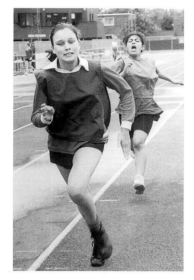

The aims of treatment should be:

- to abolish symptoms and allow children to lead a full and active life at home and at school
- to restore normal lung function
- to minimise the requirement for relief medication
- to enable normal growth and development and avoid adverse effects of medication.

These can be achieved by prompt diagnosis, identification of trigger factors, evaluation of severity, establishment of a partnership of management with the asthmatic child and the family, and regular review.

Partnership in management

Assessment of management

* Frequency of cough/wheeze
* Use of relief medication
* Days off school/activity
* Inhaler technique
* Understanding of treatment

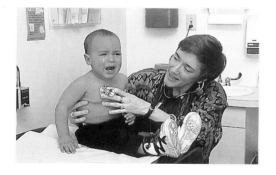

There has been much discussion recently about "self management" and "self management plans." The term is slightly misleading and a better description is partnership in management. The aim is to develop a strategy for management which will help asthmatic children and their families to cope with the day to day care of their asthma. The strategy should be adapted to the severity of the asthma and to the home and school circumstances. Partnership in management comprises:

- understanding asthma and its treatment
- monitoring symptoms
- if the child is old enough, use of a peak flow meter,
- an agreed action plan of what to do if the asthma improves, gets worse or the child has an acute asthma attack
- written guidelines.

Trained respiratory nurses working in asthma clinics and in schools have a vital role in partnership management. There are also many educational aids available including written material produced by lay organisations such as the National Asthma Campaign, videos, computer programs, and so on. They are valuable supplements to but not substitutes for regular personal contact between families and appropriately trained healthcare professionals.

Changing the environment

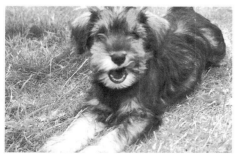

Irresistible but not desirable in asthmatic families.

The avoidance of cigarette smoke is important. Families with asthmatic children should be encouraged not to acquire pets. Pets have to go when allergy has been clearly established, but it may be months before the dander disappears completely from dust in the home. One must be quite sure that a household pet really is triggering the asthma before advising its removal because the resulting emotional upset could make things worse. When assessing allergy the history is important; it is not enough to rely on the results of skin tests or measurements of IgE antibodies.

House dust mite sensitivity is the most common allergy in asthmatic children. When such children live in schools at high altitudes where

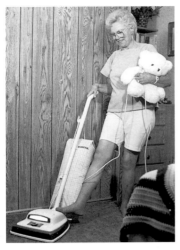

Vigorous vacuuming reduces allergens.

concentrations of house dust mite and other inhaled antigens are low, their symptoms, bronchial reactivity, and the need for medication are considerably reduced. If effective avoidance of allergens to which a child is sensitised can be achieved in the home, then the asthma will improve. Stringent measures to eradicate mites from the normal domestic environment, including removing carpets and curtains, covering mattresses, frequent laundering of bed linen, and removing soft toys have been shown to improve asthma, but such measures are difficult and time consuming.

A number of other methods which are potentially less disruptive to family life are now available. These include the application of acaricide sprays, the use of powerful filtered vacuum cleaners, and the placing of air filters and ionisers in the bedroom. The few controlled clinical trials of the use of acaricide sprays in the homes of children with asthma have given conflicting results and no acaricides are completely non-toxic, so more work needs to be done before they can be generally recommended. Vigorous vacuuming certainly reduces the allergen load. It is doubtful whether the use of a powerful (and expensive) cleaner is any better then frequent vacuuming with a conventional machine, but the incorporation of a filter may well be advantageous. Air filters and ionisers have not been shown to improve asthma.

DRUG TREATMENT

Guidelines are now available for the treatment of asthma.

Recent national and international guidelines for the management of childhood asthma have proposed a stepwise or algorithmic approach to drug management choosing a treatment regimen based on the initial assessment and then moving up or down according to the response.

Bronchodilators

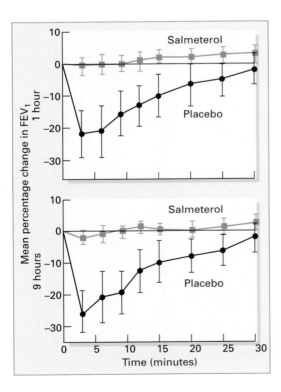

Children with mild episodic asthma need only intermittent treatment with bronchodilator drugs which should be given whenever possible by inhalation (step 1). Those with more severe asthma who are taking a prophylactic agent should always have a fast acting bronchodilator readily available. The selective β_2–adrenergic agonists (for example, salbutamol and terbutaline) are the best and safest bronchodilators. Asthma in childhood is often triggered by viral respiratory tract infections and exercise. It may be necessary to take a bronchodilator regularly during and for a week or two after a "cold." If the bronchodilator has to be continued for longer, treatment with a prophylactic agent should be considered. A single dose of an inhaled β–adrenergic bronchodilator taken 15–20 minutes before a games period at school helps to prevent exercise–induced wheezing.

In wheezy infants β-adrenergic bronchodilators inhaled through a nebuliser are often ineffective and may sometimes be associated with worsening of intrathoracic airway function: the poor response may be related to the small dose of drug reaching the airways. One study of a spacer device specifically designed for use in babies showed consistent improvement in lung function after salbutamol. In young children the anticholinergic agent ipratropium bromide may also be beneficial given either through a nebuliser or a spacer device with a face mask.

The recent development of inhaled, long acting β–adrenergic bronchodilators has added a new dimension to asthma treatment. Salmeterol is licensed for use in children from the age of 4 years. It increases the calibre of the airway for at least 12 hours and one dose prevents exercise–induced asthma for at least 9 hours. The safety profile is similar to that of salbutamol. Although symptoms improve when salmeterol is given alone it is generally agreed that it is more appropriate to use it in conjunction with regular anti-inflammatory treatment (steps 4–5). Its long duration of action makes it particularly suitable for treating nocturnal symptoms. It also has a potentially important place in the treatment of children with troublesome exercise induced asthma. Given as a single dose in the morning it will help protect against activity–induced asthma throughout the day.

Prophylactic agents

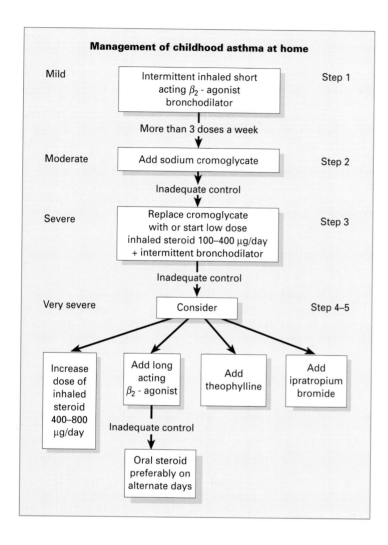

Management of childhood asthma at home

Mild — Intermittent inhaled short acting β_2 - agonist bronchodilator — Step 1

More than 3 doses a week ↓

Moderate — Add sodium cromoglycate — Step 2

Inadequate control ↓

Severe — Replace cromoglycate with or start low dose inhaled steroid 100–400 µg/day + intermittent bronchodilator — Step 3

Inadequate control ↓

Very severe — Consider — Step 4–5

Increase dose of inhaled steroid 400–800 µg/day

Add long acting β_2 - agonist

Add theophylline

Add ipratropium bromide

Inadequate control ↓

Oral steroid preferably on alternate days

Indications for prescribing inhaled steroids for children

- Moderate asthma not adequately controlled by cromoglycate
- When it is not possible to give a drug 3–4 times/day (step 2–3)
- When asthma is more severe (step 3 or 4)

Indications

The following are indications to give regular prophylactic medication:

- Symptoms and the need to take a bronchodilator several days a week.
- Frequent nocturnal cough and wheezing even without troublesome asthma during the day
- At least one asthma attack a month
- Failure of lung function to return to normal between attacks.

Lung function between attacks can be assessed by spirometric measurements of forced expiratory volume in one second (FEV1) and forced vital capacity (FVC). More subtle abnormalities can be detected by forced expiratory flow volume curves or by measurement of lung volumes in a respiratory function laboratory. A single measurement of peak expiratory flow rate (PEFR) may be misleading, but recordings made at home in the morning and evening over a week or two may show variations in PEFR that indicate airway instability and the need for prophylactic medication. Once started, regular treatment with a prophylactic agent is likely to be needed for years rather than months and should be withdrawn only when there has been little need for bronchodilator treatment for at least three months. Close supervision is necessary during withdrawal of a prophylactic drug.

Sodium cromoglycate

Despite its prolonged use in childhood and adult asthma, the exact mode of action of sodium cromoglycate remains unknown. Both British and international guidelines recommend cromoglycate as the first line preventive agent for children with moderate asthma (step 2). Taken regularly it will control asthma in about 60% of school age children with frequent symptoms. The metered dose aerosol is as effective as the powder in children who are able to use it properly and is slightly less likely to cause coughing after inhalation. Nebulised cromoglycate improves asthma in preschool children. It does not reduce hospital admission rates or severe wheezing provoked by viral respiratory infections, and appears to be ineffective in wheezy infants. The reduction in efficacy when cromoglycate is given by nebuliser to very young children may be because at this age only a small amount of the drug reaches the airways.

Sodium cromoglycate is completely safe with virtually no side effects even when taken regularly for years, which is a strong argument for using it when possible. Unfortunately the requirement for it to be taken three or four times a day makes non-compliance a common reason for failure of treatment. Sodium cromoglycate is unlikely to control symptoms in children with severe asthma. The response to cromoglycate should be carefully evaluated 2–3 months after starting treatment and it is important to decide whether optimal control of asthma has been achieved or merely some improvement in symptoms. If the asthma is still interfering with the child's daily activity, if the peak flow is unstable, or if the child still requires frequent relief medication, cromoglycate should be replaced by a low dose of an inhaled steroid (step 3).

Inhaled steroids

Corticosteroids are the most potent anti-inflammatory agents available

Asthma in children: treatment

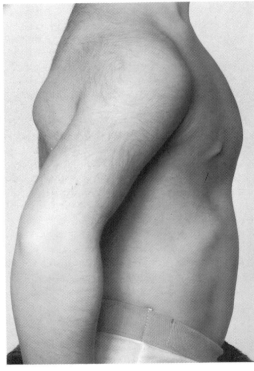

Chest deformity like this is an indication to treat with inhaled steroids.

for treating asthma, and they have the greatest diversity of action. Indications for prescribing inhaled steroids to children are:

- moderate asthma which is not adequately controlled by cromoglycate
- when it is not possible to give a drug 3–4 times a day (step 2 to step 3)
- when asthma is more severe (step 3 or step 4).

The presence of chest deformity is an absolute indication to treat with an inhaled steroid. The starting dose depends on the clinical assessment of severity but in children with frequent symptoms there are theoretical reasons for starting with a relatively high dose (400–800 μg/day) and reducing the dose once the asthma comes under control.

Inhaled steroids given by pressurised aerosol or by powder inhaler are effective in older children. Combining an inhaled steroid with cromoglycate does not confer additional benefit. In recent years inhaled steroids have been used increasingly to treat preschool asthma. When an inhaled steroid is given to pre-school children with frequent or severe asthma through a large volume spacer with a one way valve or mask it is as effective as it is in older children, and this seems to be the best delivery system for the very young. Trials of steroids given by nebuliser to young children in conventional doses (200–400 μg/day) have given disappointing results. This is almost certainly because the amount of drug delivered in a suspension from a nebuliser to a freely breathing infant or young child is small. Over three quarters of the inhaled steroid remains in the nebuliser and fewer than 20% of the nebulised droplets containing drug are less than 5 μm in diameter. To overcome this problem it is necessary to use large starting doses. Trials of budesonide 1000 to 2000 μg/day have shown a therapeutic effect in infants with severe asthma.

Understandably there is a reluctance to give inhaled steroids to young children because of concern about possible side effects. Local side effects such as oral thrush and dysphonia are rare in childhood probably because powder inhalers and spacer devices are used. Inhaled steroids have a dose dependent effect on the adrenal glands by which they reduce resting cortisol output. There is no evidence, however, that inhaled steroids given to children in doses of up to 400 μg/day cause clinically important suppression of the hypothalamus-pituitary-adrenal axis. The effect of inhaled steroids on growth is difficult to assess because any possible effect will interact with the effect on growth of the disease itself. Inhaled steroids in high doses—particularly when given by powder inhaler—sometimes cause growth deceleration. On the other hand poor asthma control has a much greater adverse effect on growth than inhaled corticosteroids and control of severe asthma by treatment with an inhaled steroid often leads to an acceleration in height velocity.

Not all inhaled steroids are the same. There is evidence that in high doses budesonide has less effect on the hypothalamus-pituitary-adrenal axis than beclomethasone dipropionate and that fluticasone propionate has lower systemic bioavailability than either beclomethasone or budesonide.

Oral agents

When a drug has to be taken regularly there are obvious advantages if it can be taken by mouth and only twice a day.

Slow release theophyllines in doses titrated to give blood concentrations of 10–20 mg/l will control asthma in about 60% of children with frequent symptoms but they are relatively ineffective in preventing the wheezing which accompanies viral upper respiratory tract infections. The variable clearance rate of theophylline in children means that it is difficult to predict the dose of the drug that will give "therapeutic" blood concentrations in an individual child. Side effects (notably gastointestinal upsets and behaviour disturbances) are common particularly in preschool children. Because of problems with giving the drug and its side effects the use of theophyllines has been restricted to children whose asthma is uncontrolled despite treatment with inhaled steroids (steps 4–5).

Inhaler devices

Children should be treated with inhalers if possible.

Whenever possible asthma treatment should be given to children by inhalation, and the most common reasons for failure of inhaled treatment are inappropriate selection or incorrect use of the inhaler. Children become fully aware of their own breathing and recognise the difference between inspiration and expiration by about the age of 3 years; until then they need inhalation devices which require only tidal breathing. Inspiratory flow rates are slower and the airways narrower in children and both these factors influence the dose inhaled and the site of deposition of the drug. The choice of inhaler will depend on the child's age and on the family's preference for a particular device.

Inhaler devices for children

	Relief	Prevention
0–2 years		
Large volume spacer + face mask*	Ipratropium Salbutamol Terbutaline	Cromoglycate Beclomethasone Budesonide
Coffee cup*	Ipratropium Salbutamol Terbutaline	
Nebuliser	Ipratropium Salbutamol Terbutaline	Cromoglycate Budesonide
3–4 years		
Large volume spacer*	Salbutamol Terbutaline	Cromoglycate Beclomethasone Budesonide
5 years and over		
Autohaler	Salbutamol	Beclomethasone
Diskhaler/rotahaler	Salbutamol Salmeterol	Fluticasone Beclomethasone
Spinhaler		Cromoglycate
Turbohaler	Terbutaline	Budesonide

* Metered dose inhaler

Aerosols and powders

Most children under the age of 10 years are unable to achieve the coordination needed to use an unmodified metered dose aerosol inhaler. Less than half the children obtain benefit from these devices because of poor inhalation technique. Breath actuated metered dose inhalers (Autohaler) are easier to use but a child tends to close the glottis when the breath actuated valve opens and the number that are able to use these inhalers declines rapidly under the age of 7 years.

Breath actuated powder inhalers are either single dose (Spinhaler, Rotahaler) or multiple dose (Diskhaler, Tubuhaler). The multiple dose inhalers are easier to use but it is more difficult to monitor the number of doses taken. The age at which breath actuated powder inhalers can be used depends on the optimal inspiratory flow rate: for example the Rotahaler requires a inspiration of at least 90 l/minute whereas the Turbuhaler needs an inspiration of about 30 l/minute. The latter can therefore be used in younger children.

Spacers and nebulisers

A spacer device reduces the velocity of the particles before they reach the mouth and allows more of the propellent to evaporate so that the inhaled particles become smaller and penetrate further into the lungs. After activation of the drug cannister, the aerosol can be inhaled by taking a few breaths sufficient to open and close the valve attached to the mouthpiece. Children can use large volume spacers in this way from the age of 2 years. If the spacer is turned upside down so that the valve falls open and a mask is attached to the mouthpiece, it can be used to give asthma treatment to infants. During acute asthma attacks young children may not be able to move the valve in which case only nebulised treatment is appropriate.

Nebulisers are expensive, time consuming, and inconvenient and they are often used incorrectly at home. A compressor and jet nebuliser suitable for giving asthma medication should have a driving gas flow rate of 8–10 l/minute and a volume fill of 4 ml; this is particularly important when giving a suspension such as an inhaled steroid. It is not justified to assume that the equivalent dose for older children is appropriate for a younger age group because inhalation technique, tidal volume breathing, and the anatomy of the upper airway are different. Despite these reservations, however, there is an important place for the judicious use of nebulisers in the treatment of young asthmatic children at home.

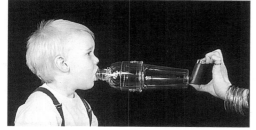

A child using a large volume spacer with assistance.

ACUTE SEVERE ASTHMA

Some indications for hospital admission

Signs	Cyanosis
	Exhaustion
	Difficulty in speaking
	Pulsus paradoxus >20 mm
Peak flow rate	<25% of predicted
Response	No improvement despite adequate doses of inhaled bronchodilator
Experience	Known pattern of attacks

Parents and children need clear instructions about what to do when an acute asthma attack occurs and when to ask for medical help. If the attack does not respond quickly to the child's usual relief medication, treatment should be given with a large dose of a β-stimulant bronchodilator (salbutamol, terbutaline) by nebuliser or large volume spacer. Subcutaneous terbutaline 0.005 mg (0.01 ml)/kg is less satisfactory because of the distress caused by the injection. Consideration should be given to starting oral prednisolone. The response to treatment should be documented objectively in all children old enough to use a peak flow meter. A child who responds well to a high dose of nebulised bronchodilator at home will need to be reviewed a few hours later, and will require increased treatment for a week or more afterwards.

The principles of assessment and treatment in hospital of children over the age of 18 months are similar to those for adults. When faced with an intravenous infusion young children sometimes become extremely distressed and make their asthma worse, in which case it may be better to treat them with nebulised salbutamol, ipratropium bromide, and oral steroids.

Oxygen is important in treatment but sometimes difficult to give to toddlers. They become dehydrated because of poor fluid intake, sweating, and—in the early stages—hyperventilation. This must be corrected, but there are potential risks of overhydrating children with severe asthma. Production of antidiuretic hormone may be increased during the attack, and the considerable negative intrathoracic pressures generated by the respiratory efforts may predispose to pulmonary oedema. After correcting dehydration the wisest course is to give normal fluid requirements and measure the plasma and urine osmolality.

A child should not be discharged from hospital until he is taking the treatment that he will be taking at home, and on this treatment the peak flow rate should be at least 75% of expected.

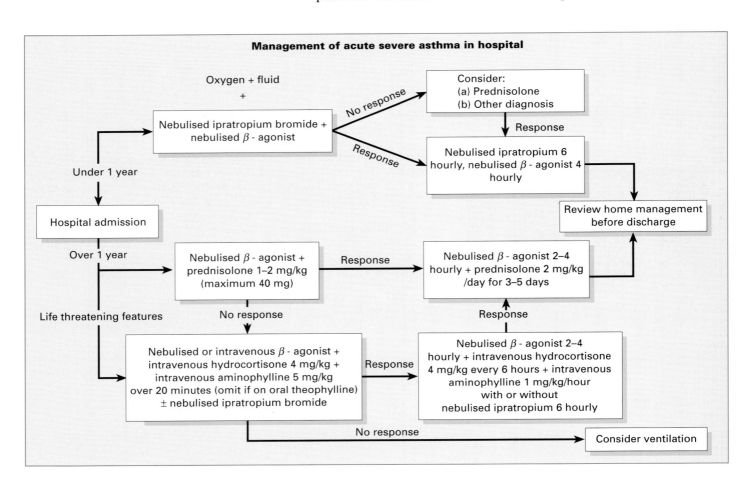

46

INDEX

Index

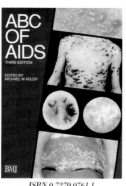

ABC OF AIDS
THIRD EDITION
EDITED BY
MICHAEL W ADLER
BMJ

ISBN 0 7279 0761 1

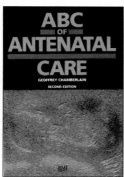

ABC OF ANTENATAL CARE
GEOFFREY CHAMBERLAIN
SECOND EDITION
BMJ

ISBN 0 7279 0884 7

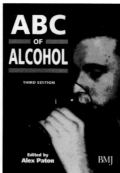

ABC OF SLEEP DISORDERS
Edited by
Colin M Shapiro
BMJ

ISBN 0 7279 0794 8

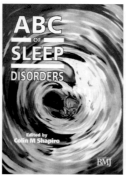

ABC OF ALCOHOL
THIRD EDITION
Edited by
Alex Paton
BMJ

ISBN 0 7279 0812 X

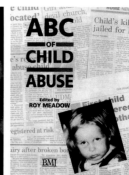

ABC OF CHILD ABUSE
Edited by
ROY MEADOW
BMJ

ISBN 0 7279 0764 6

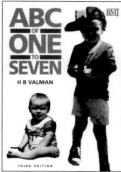

ABC OF ONE TO SEVEN
H B VALMAN
THIRD EDITION

ISBN 0 7279 0768 9

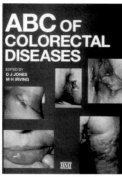

ABC OF COLORECTAL DISEASES
EDITED BY
D J JONES
M H IRVING
BMJ

ISBN 0 7279 0755 7

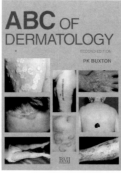

ABC OF DERMATOLOGY
SECOND EDITION
PK BUXTON
BMJ

ISBN 0 7279 0777 8

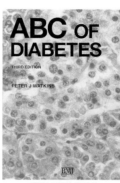

ABC OF DIABETES
THIRD EDITION
PETER J WATKINS
BMJ

ISBN 0 7279 0763 8

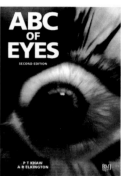

ABC OF EYES
SECOND EDITION
P T KHAW
A R ELKINGTON
BMJ

ISBN 0 7279 0766 2

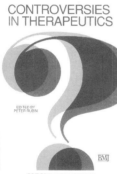

CONTROVERSIES IN THERAPEUTICS
?
EDITED BY
PETER RUBIN
BMJ

ISBN 0 7279 0299 7

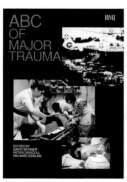

ABC OF MAJOR TRAUMA
BMJ
EDITED BY
DAVID SKINNER
PETER DRISCOLL
RICHARD EARLAM
BMJ

ISBN 0 7279 0291 1

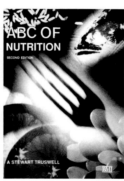

ABC OF NUTRITION
SECOND EDITION
A STEWART TRUSWELL
BMJ

ISBN 0 7279 0315 2

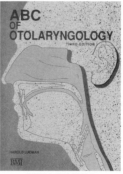

ABC OF OTOLARYNGOLOGY
THIRD EDITION
HAROLD LUDMAN
BMJ

ISBN 0 7279 0765 4

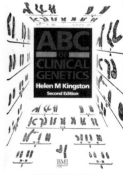

ABC OF CLINICAL GENETICS
Helen M Kingston
Second Edition
BMJ

ISBN 0 7279 0846 4

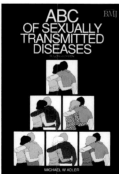

ABC OF SEXUALLY TRANSMITTED DISEASES
SECOND EDITION
MICHAEL W ADLER
BMJ

ISBN 0 7279 0261 X

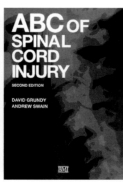

ABC OF SPINAL CORD INJURY
SECOND EDITION
DAVID GRUNDY
ANDREW SWAIN
BMJ

ISBN 0 7279 0760 3

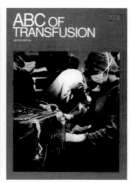

ABC OF TRANSFUSION
SECOND EDITION
BMJ

ISBN 0 7279 0754 9

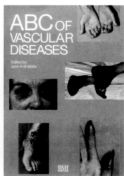

ABC OF VASCULAR DISEASES
Edited by
John H N Wolfe
BMJ

ISBN 0 7279 0259 8

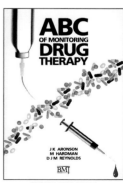

ABC OF MONITORING DRUG THERAPY
J K ARONSON
M HARDMAN
D J M REYNOLDS
BMJ

ISBN 0 7279 0791 3

For further details contact your local bookseller or write to:

Books Division
BMJ Publishing Group
BMA House
Tavistock Square
London WC1H 9JR (U.K.)

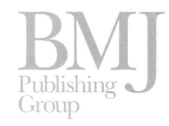

BMJ Publishing Group